Praise for *Introduction to Autonomic Medicine*:

This book is an excellent resource for clinicians, students, and researchers of human physiology and related fields. Dr. Goldstein provides descriptions and illustrations that are easy to grasp and easy to remember. The text will become a dog-eared favorite in many libraries.

Glen Cook, MD, Director, Autonomic Disorders Clinic
at Walter Reed National Military Medical Center
Course Director, *The Residents Course Advancing Autonomic Medicine*

This foundational text is a must-read for those interested in the autonomic nervous system. Dr. Goldstein introduces topics with clear illustrations,and follows with a rich exploration of more complex concepts. There is something for everyone in this book, from students to practicing clinicians, scientifically minded patients, and even advanced autonomic specialists looking to hone their teaching of the subject.

Elisabeth Golden, MD, Neurohospitalist specializing in
neuromuscular and autonomic disorders, UT Health Tyler
Faculty, *The Residents Course Advancing Autonomic Medicine*

Introduction to Autonomic Medicine is a foundational textbook. Dr. Goldstein is a world-renowned expert who has influenced generations of autonomic specialists and scientists. The book is a testament to his ability to distill incredibly complicated information into memorable, digestible, and clinically relevant points. I will recommend it to house staff, students, faculty, and scientists who wish to gain a deep understanding of autonomic science and medicine.

Nathaniel M. Robbins MD, Harvard Medical School
Director, MGH/Brigham Program
in Small Fiber and Autonomic Neurology
Faculty, *The Residents Course Advancing Autonomic Medicine*

I was fortunate to attend Dr. Goldstein's lecture in *The Residents Course Advancing Autonomic Medicine*. After reading the book, I was once again impressed by his comprehensive knowledge of the autonomic system, from fundamental biochemistry and neuroanatomy to clinical applications. The book explains concepts clearly and includes vivid metaphors that make reading enjoyable. As a neurologist, I anticipate using it frequently as a reference in my future practice.

Dr. Yuanyuan Tan,
Texas Tech University Health Sciences Center
PGY4 Neurology Residency Program
The Residents Course Graduate, 2024

To the memory of

David Robertson, MD (1947-2024)

He founded the first center of excellence focused on autonomic disorders at Vanderbilt University Medical Center in 1979. The first informal meeting of the American Autonomic Society (AAS) took place in his living room in Nashville, Tennessee in 1990. A pioneer in autonomic medicine, he spent over 30 years pursuing rigorous research in the field. He trained several generations of mentees many of whom are leaders in autonomic medicine today. Those who knew him—colleagues, mentees, and patients—remember his soft-spoken kindness, humility, and genuine dedication to the care of people.

INTRODUCTION TO AUTONOMIC MEDICINE

ISBN 978-1938842-67-2

For inquiries, please contact *info@DysProject.org*.

Published by Bardolf & Company
www.bardolfandcompany.com

Cover Design by Autumn Kerr of Cultivate Place Creative

Introduction to

AUTONOMIC MEDICINE

David S. Goldstein, MD PhD

Edited and Foreword by
Kelly Freeman, MSM

Bardolf & Company
Sarasota, Florida

CONTENTS

Disclaimer

About the Author

Dr. David S. Goldstein is an internationally recognized authority and clincal researcher in autonomic medicine. He graduated in 1970 from Yale College and completed an MD/PhD at Johns Hopkins in 1976. He has been a tenured Senior Investigator in intramural programs of the National Institutes of Health (NIH) since 1984. In 1990 he came to the National Institute of Neurological Disorders and Stroke (NINDS), where he has served as Chief of the Clinical Neurochemistry Section, the Clinical Neurocardiology Section, and the Autonomic Medicine Section. His main discovery is cardiac sympathetic denervation in Lewy body diseases such as Parkinson's disease.

To date he has more than 650 publications, which have been cited more than 50,000 times, including more than 135 cited more than 100 times each. Among his honors are the Society for Clinical and Translational Science's Distinguished Investigator Award, the American Academy of Neurology's Irwin Schatz Award in Autonomic Disorders, the NIH Distinguished Clinical Teacher Award, 2 NINDS Director's Awards, election to the Association of American Physicians, and the Johns Hopkins School of Medicine Distinguished Medical Alumnus Award. His single-authored e-textbook, Principles of Autonomic Medicine, is a unique resource available for free download from his NINDS webpage. His main strategic goals are to establish autonomic medicine as a clinical and scientific discipline, promote patient-oriented research on autonomic and catecholamine-related disorders, and mentor rising investigators in the field.

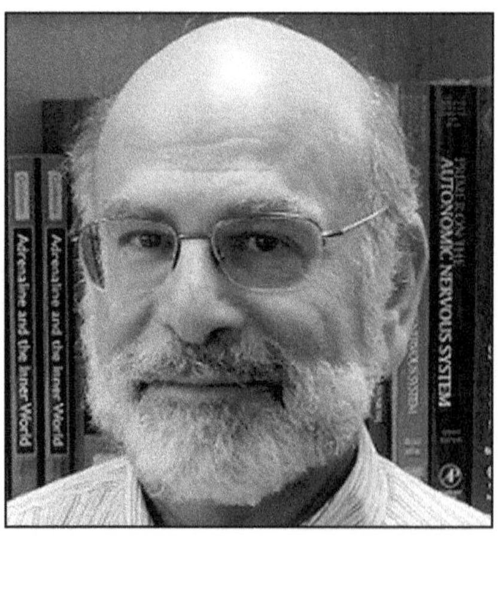

About the Editor

Kelly Freeman is founder of the Dysautonomia Project, a 501c3 nonprofit organization created to educate patients and healthcare providers around the world about autonomic disorders. She is also co-author of the award-winning *Dysautonomia Project* book. In collaboration with the American Autonomic Society, she has created free online courses in autonomic medicine (AutonomicEducation.com). She has also helped to establish several courses in autonomic education including *The Residents Course*, a mini-fellowship in autonomic medicine, *The Clinician Program*, a one day course for providers, and *DysCourse*, an annual program for patients and caregivers. For more information about these programs visit *www.DysProject.org*.

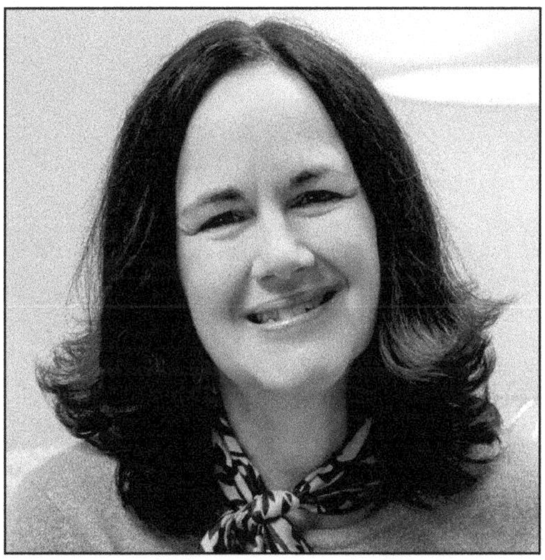

FOREWORD

Kelly Freeman, MSM

I am excited to bring this book to you at a time when autonomic medicine is emerging across the globe as an important subspecialty in healthcare.

The overwhelming majority of medicine today is based on the assumption that a patient's autonomic nervous system is intact and functioning normally. But what if it is not? What do we do when there are abnormalities in the body's regulatory functions, such as maintaining normal blood flow to the heart, lungs, and brain while standing upright, or sweating properly to keep cool on a hot day? *Introduction to Autonomic Medicine* is the starting point for understanding the crucial role the autonomic nervous system plays in all of healthcare.

The author, David S. Goldstein, is the most internationally recognized and most published expert on the topic. In an easy-to-understand way, he discusses the workings of the autonomic nervous system, various tests of autonomic function, and disorders of the autonomic nervous system. He also created more than 100 illustrations to make this textbook a useful resource for:

- Medical students, residents, or fellows
- Practicing clinicians, nurses, and other health care providers
- Scientists and researchers
- Patients who want a more scientific understanding of dysautonomias

I first met David Goldstein ten years ago at a meeting where he used a flipchart to draw pictures as he taught about many ideas contained in this book. First, he drew a tootsie roll pop analogous to the design of the central nervous system. Then, he drew the chemical structure of a catecholamine and taught us to remember that catecholamines look like cats. As he lectured, I thought he is not only one of the world's top academic scientists in autonomic medicine, but also a gifted and creative teacher.

At that time, I was looking for a few well-respected doctors of autonomic medicine who might be willing to help me educate others about dysautonomias by helping me write a book for both patients and healthcare providers. I was thrilled when David offered to help me co-author *The Dysautonomia Project*.

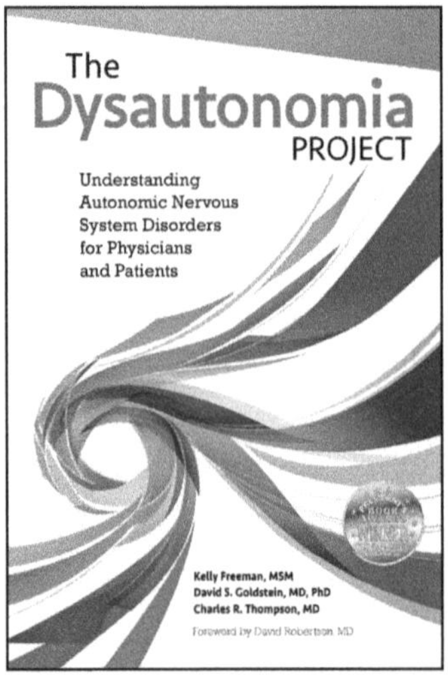

While working with him on that book, I learned the importance of ensuring that everything we teach is science-based and backed by research. David never hesitated to correct or challenge a thought in the name of scientific accuracy. Since then, we have collaborated on several projects, including the free online video library created by the American Autonomic Society (AAS) and The Dysautonomia Project (TDP), which includes the course, *Introduction to Autonomic Medicine*, and gave this book its name.

At the outset, the idea was to create a textbook for *The Residents Course*, a mini-fellowship advancing autonomic medicine for medical residents. We envisioned a shortened version of David's *Principles of Autonomic Medicine*, a 734-page, free online, full-color textbook. While many people have viewed and referenced the online book, its sheer size makes it difficult to use as a teaching tool. I may have been one of the few who downloaded and printed the whole thing.

With time, it became clear that this version of the book is not just for medical residents or trainees—it is a starting point for every current and future health care provider in understanding the important role the autonomic nervous system plays in the human body. And for healthcare providers, it is also the next step in learning after reading *The Dysautonomia Project* book.

I have been fortunate to witness David's passion for education, which has helped to shape the study of autonomic medicine over the past decade. I believe his work on this topic will be a significant reference for generations to come.

Introduction to

AUTONOMIC MEDICINE

This book has the goal of teaching residents, medical students, clinicians, nurses, and others about autonomic disorders.

INTRODUCTION

Why Are Dysautonomias Hard?

Dysautonomias are a difficult subject for patients, doctors, students, and researchers. Dysautonomias are hard to diagnose, treat, live with, and understand. There are several reasons for this. It's important to explain at the outset why the field of dysautonomias is so hard.

(1) Dysautonomias are multi-disciplinary

The field of dysautonomias spans multiple disciplines of medicine. Specialists within these disciplines often cannot serve dysautonomia patients.

Cardiology (heart rhythm & rate problems, heart failure, hypertension)
Neurology (seizures, Parkinson's disease, Chiari malformation, neuropathy)
Endocrinology (diabetes, thyroid problems, adrenal problems)
Gastroenterology (esophageal problems, irritable bowel, constipation)
Psychiatry (depression, anxiety, conversion reaction)
Pediatrics (fainting, inherited/congenital disease, POTS)
Pain Medicine (migraine, fibromyalgia, neuropathic pain, TMJ disorder)
Immunology (Sjogren's, auto-immune disorders, MCAS, lupus)

Dysautonomias are hard, because they are multi-disciplinary.

If your only tool is a hammer, the world looks like a nail. If a dysautonomia patient sees a cardiologist, the cardiologist looks for an abnormal heart rhythm or heart block, something a pacemaker or ablative therapy can treat. If the patient sees a neurologist, the neurologist looks for a seizure disorder, a problem with blood flow to the brain, a brain structural abnormality, or a neuropathy. If the patient sees an endocrinologist, the endocrinologist looks for diabetes or a thyroid, adrenal, or pituitary problem. If the patient sees an immunologist, the immunologist looks for autoimmunity or mast cell activation. If the patient sees a gastroenterologist, the gastroenterologist looks for gastro-esophageal reflux, decreased gut motility, or irritable bowel syndrome. If as often happens the patient finally sees a psychiatrist, the psychiatrist looks for depression, anxiety, a "conversion reaction," or panic disorder.

(2) Dysautonomias are complex

Many factors determine levels of pulse rate, blood pressure, body metabolism, pain, fatigue, and the sense of psychological well-being. These factors interact complexly with each other.

Further complicating the picture, patients with dysautonomias often are treated with multiple drugs, which not only can interact with each other but also with the disorders. Scientific theories taking this complexity into account have lagged behind.

Diagrams depicting disorders of feedback-regulated systems can appear dauntingly complex. At their core, though, they all involve abnormal functioning of negative feedback loops.

This book teaches that dysautonomias are usually if not always disorders of integration, of regulation, of systems that change during life as a function of the balance of wear and tear vs. resilience.

(3) Different centers have different emphases

Academic and medical referral centers differ in the workup and management of dysautonomias. One center traditionally has focused on familial dysautonomia, a rare pediatric disease. Another has emphasized dysautonomia associated with diabetes, another disorders of sweating, another chronic orthostatic intolerance and multiple system atrophy, and another autoimmune autonomic ganglionopathy.

In almost every aspect of autonomic medical practice and research, doctors—even experts in the field—can disagree about answers to key questions. How should dysautonomias be classified? What are the types and subtypes? Of what do patients with particular dysautonomias complain? Which tests are useful to diagnose particular dysautonomias or monitor responses to treatments? What are the disease mechanisms? Which treatments work for which forms of dysautonomia? What happens to patients with dysautonomias over time?

Different centers offer different tests, often depending on factors such as finances, insurance coverage, regulatory constraints, and delays. In my opinion these aspects have impeded the efficient adoption and application of valuable, powerful clinical laboratory technologies.

In particular, no center outside the NIH has an integrated program of autonomic neuroimaging and neurochemistry. Tests that are done at the NIH for research purposes are not approved by the FDA as diagnostic tests.

(4) Difficult pronunciations & abbreviations

The word, "dysautonomia," is difficult to pronounce. So are the words, "norepinephrine" and "acetylcholine," which are the key chemical messengers of the autonomic nervous system.

Dysautonomias			Catecholamines		
Diss-auto-NO-mias			Cat-a-COAL-a-means		
POTS	DOPA	PPI	NE	QSART	COMT
TLOC	SSRI	DOPAC	EPI	SST	MAO
COI	NET	HSAN	DHPG	SEC	SEC
CAF	PET	CCHS	PET	MAP	DAN
PAF	F-DA	SAI	MIBG	HRV	DBH
FD	LBD	CO	DAT	ALDH	EDS
MSA	DLB	TPR	AAG	LAAAD	ILBD
PD	nOH	SV	NIDDM	VMAT	RBD
DOPS	OH	FVR	NSRI	ANS	PNS

The field of autonomic medicine is rife with abbreviations that only an expert can comprehend.

(5) Dysautonomias are "mind-body" disorders

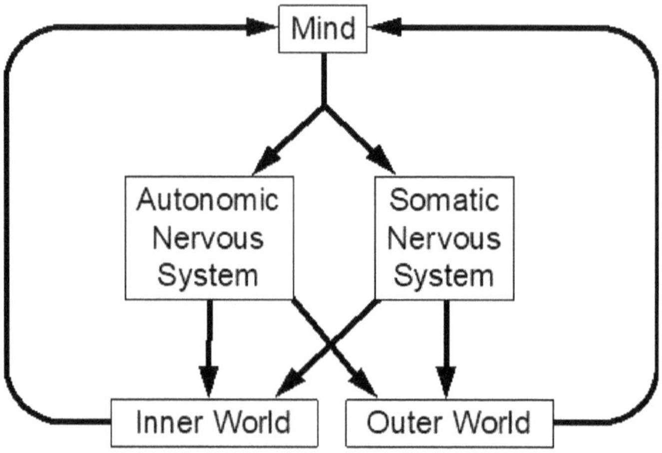

The autonomic nervous system operates at the border of the mind and body.

In this book you will learn about the "inner world" inside the body and the "outer world" outside the body. The mind deals with both worlds, simultaneously, continuously, and dynamically in life. Conversely, both worlds affect the mind, and each individual filters and colors perceptions of the inner and outer world.

For instance, there is no such thing as a person exercising without "central command," to tense and relax specific muscles. At the same time, and as part of the same process, the brain automatically directs changes in blood flow to the muscles. The exercising muscle and changes in blood flow lead to information—feedback—to the brain about how things are going both outside and inside the body.

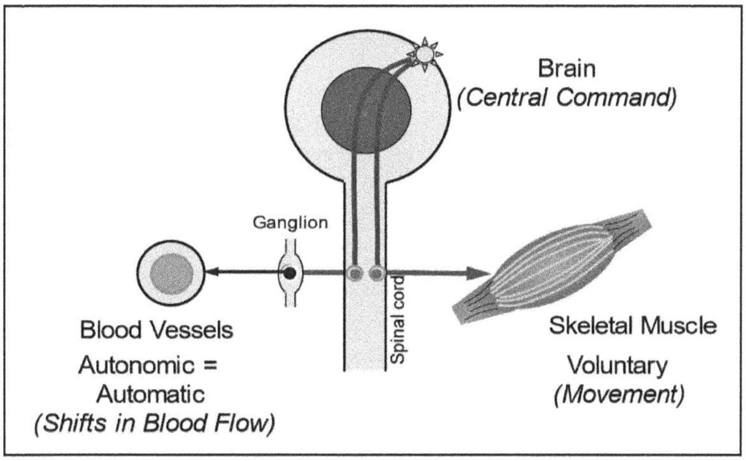

The phenomenon of "central command" involves concurrent voluntary skeletal muscle contraction and alterations in autonomic outflows to blood vessels.

A major purpose of this book is to teach that the many symptoms of dysautonomias reflect real biological or chemical changes. If a clinician cannot identify the cause of a patient's symptoms, this ignorance should not lead to dismissing the patient as having a psychiatric rather than a "real" problem. The autonomic nervous system operates exactly at the ineffable border of the mind and body. In this book you will learn a systems approach to the mind-body issue.

Are dysautonomias in the mind or body? The answer is: they are in both. The autonomic nervous system operates at the border of the mind and body.

The brain uses and depends on the autonomic nervous system for the internal adjustments that accompany every motion a person performs and every emotion a person feels. From the point of view of the bodily changes, it would matter little whether these changes resulted from the physical experience of exercise or the mental experience of rage. Both situations involve alterations in the activity of components of the autonomic nervous system. Both situations involve changes in the inner and outer worlds. And if your autonomic nervous system were to malfunction, your reactions to either situation would not be regulated correctly; in either situation you could feel sick, look sick, and be sick! A "systems" approach helps to understand dysautonomias.

According to the systems approach, the mind simultaneously directs changes in the somatic nervous system and the autonomic nervous system, based on perceptions about what is going on in the inner world and the outer world.

How would a systems approach help to understand a dysautonomia? A malfunction at almost any part of the system could lead to alterations in activities of components of the autonomic nervous system. For instance, if there were no feedback to the brain about the state of the blood pressure (part of the inner world), then there would be an inability to keep the blood pressure within bounds, by changing the activity of the sympathetic noradrenergic system. If there were no feedback about the extent of physical exercise, there would also be an inability to adjust the blood pressure and blood flows appropriately. Of course, if there were a failure of the autonomic nervous system itself, this would also interfere with regulation of the inner world, but there would also be difficulty in dealing with the outer world, manifested by problems like exercise intolerance or an inability to tolerate standing for a prolonged period (orthostatic intolerance). Finally, if the person had a psychiatric disorder such as panic/anxiety, then the inappropriate emotional experience of fear would be linked to both autonomic nervous system and somatic nervous system changes.

A clinician's ability to treat a dysautonomia successfully also benefits from a systems approach. Treatments at any of several steps might help, but the best place in the system to insert a treatment would be the step closest to where the cause is if there were only one.

(6) Dysautonomias are not taught well

The field of clinical disorders of the autonomic nervous system is taught well at any educational level. Medical and graduate school curricula rarely contain coursework on dysautonomias. Compared to the large patient demand and public health burden, clinical and basic training and scientific knowledge about dysautonomias are disproportionately sparse.

In other words, if you are reading this book, you're on the cutting edge!

WHAT IS THE ANS?

This section is about how the nervous system functions when there is nothing wrong with it. You will need to understand the basics before you can understand the problems that can develop.

To keep you alive your body has to be able to coordinate many different activities. Some of these activities are voluntary and conscious, like moving your legs to walk across the room, while others are involuntary and unconscious, like breathing and digesting.

> The autonomic nervous system (ANS) is the body's "automatic nervous system."

The ANS is responsible for many of the automatic, usually unconscious processes that keep the body alive and stable, such as:

- controlling blood flows to the brain and other organs, both while you are at rest and while you are exercising.
- keeping the right body temperature.
- digesting food for energy production and fuel delivery.
- getting rid of waste products in the urine and feces.
- generating warning signs such as sweating, turning pale, and trembling in dangerous situations.

Here is a classical diagram illustrating the organization of the ANS.

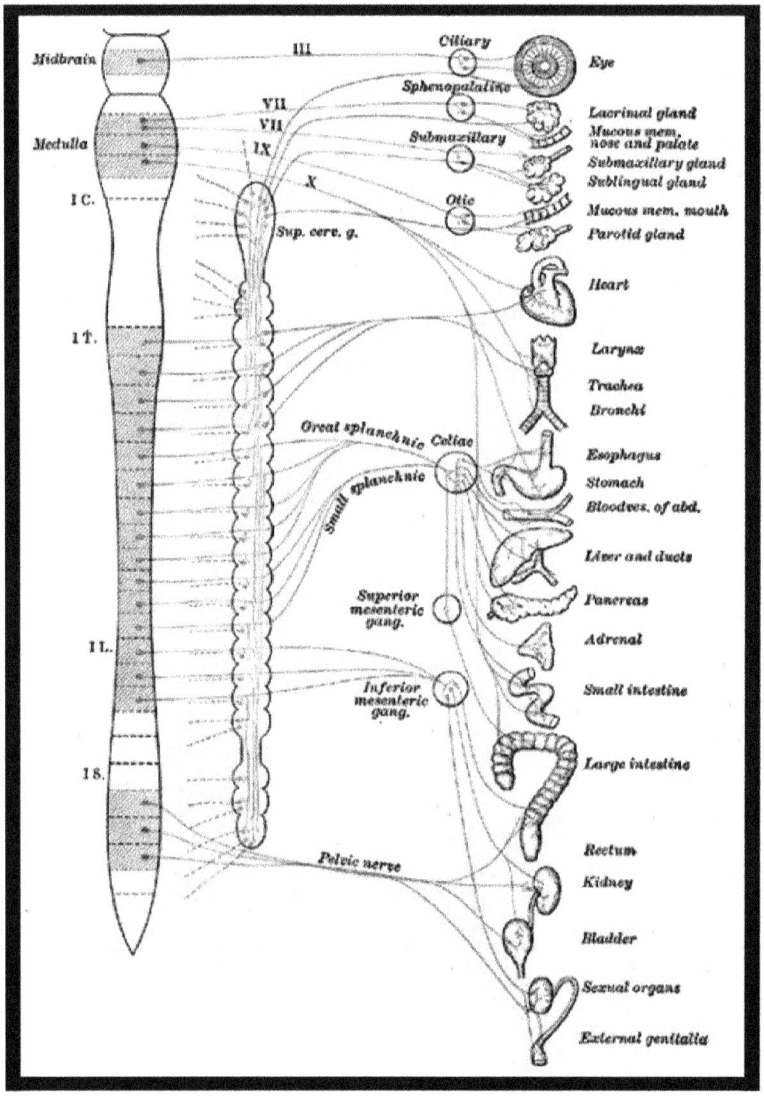

Diagram of autonomic nervous outflows to body organs.

The Tootsie Roll pop analogy

The organization of the ANS seems impossibly complex. Let's start to build up from scratch.

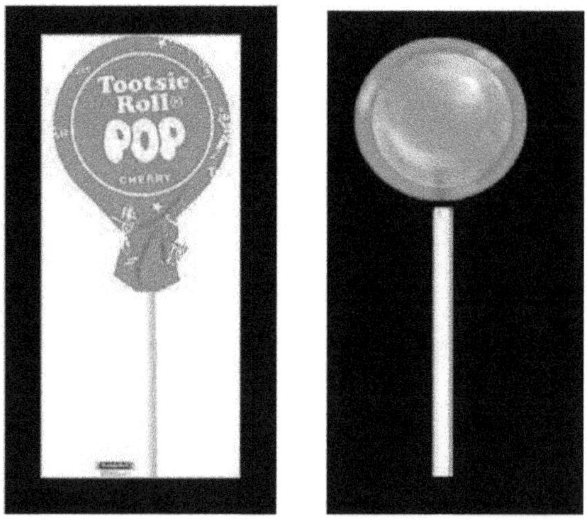

The central nervous system is like a Tootsie Roll pop. The brain is the candy. The spinal cord is the stick.

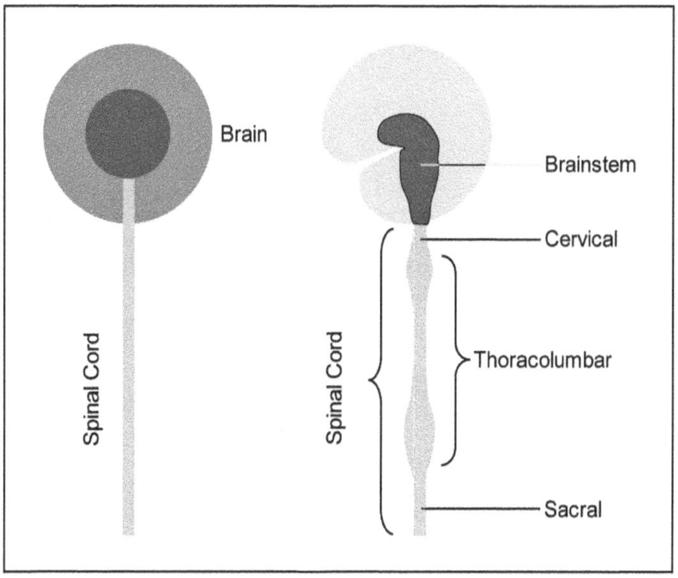

In the Tootsie Roll Pop analogy, the chewy chocolate center is the brainstem.

The central nervous system (CNS) is made up of the brain and the spinal cord. The brain is like a command and control center. The spinal cord is a rope of nerves that runs from the base of your brain down through your back within your spinal column. The spinal cord is divided up into regions or levels. The cervical spinal cord is in the neck. Below this are the thoracic and lumbar spinal cord (the two parts together are the thoracolumbar spinal cord), and the lowest level is the sacral spinal cord.

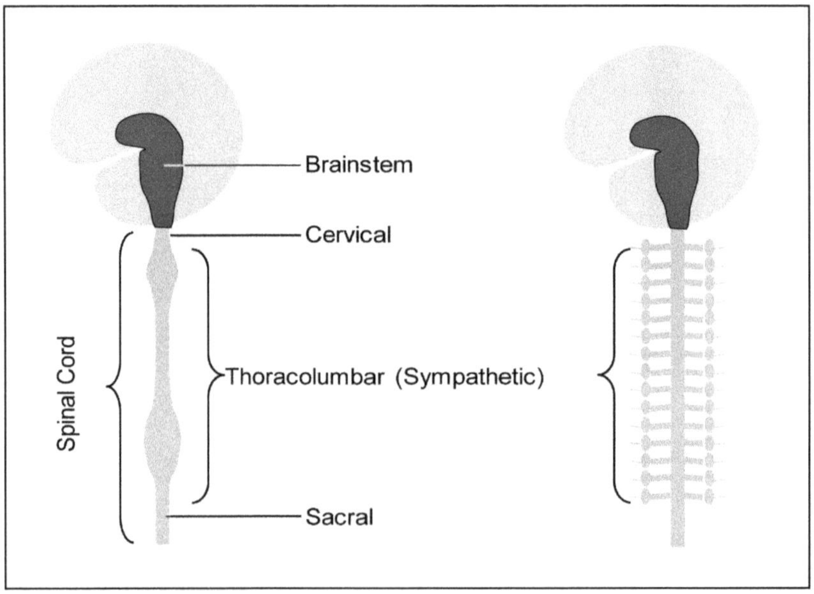

Autonomic nerves are derived from the brainstem and the thoracolumbar and sacral spinal cord.

Control signals travel from your brain to your limbs and organs by way of the peripheral nervous system. The peripheral nerves are all the nerves that lie outside the brain and spinal cord.

Ganglia: the utility pole outside your house

Nerves that travel to skeletal muscle and regulate movement come directly from the central nervous system. Nervous signals of the ANS, however, travel indirectly to internal organs, via clumps of cells called "ganglia."

As we'll discuss later, one of the major components of the ANS is the sympathetic nervous system. The ganglia of the sympathetic nervous system and connecting trunks run parallel to the spinal column. The cell bodies of the sympathetic nerves that project to body organs therefore are not in the brain or spinal cord.

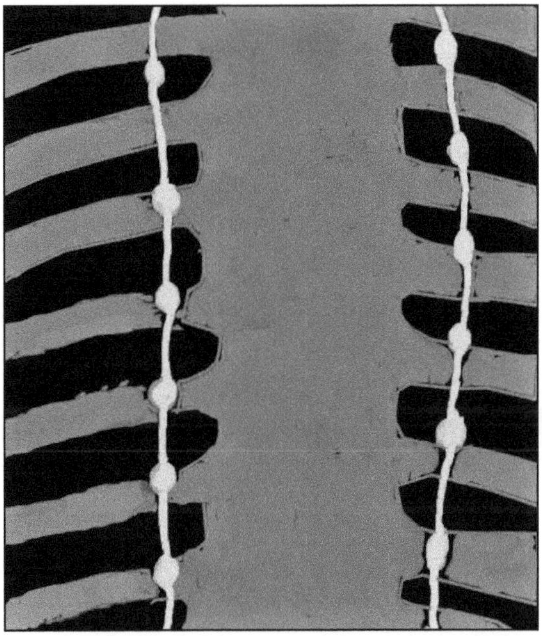

Sympathetic ganglia are arranged like pearls on a necklace on each side of the spinal column.

A way to identify the ganglia and nerve trunks connecting them is via the spinal nerves, which are thick and run perpendicular to the sympathetic chain.

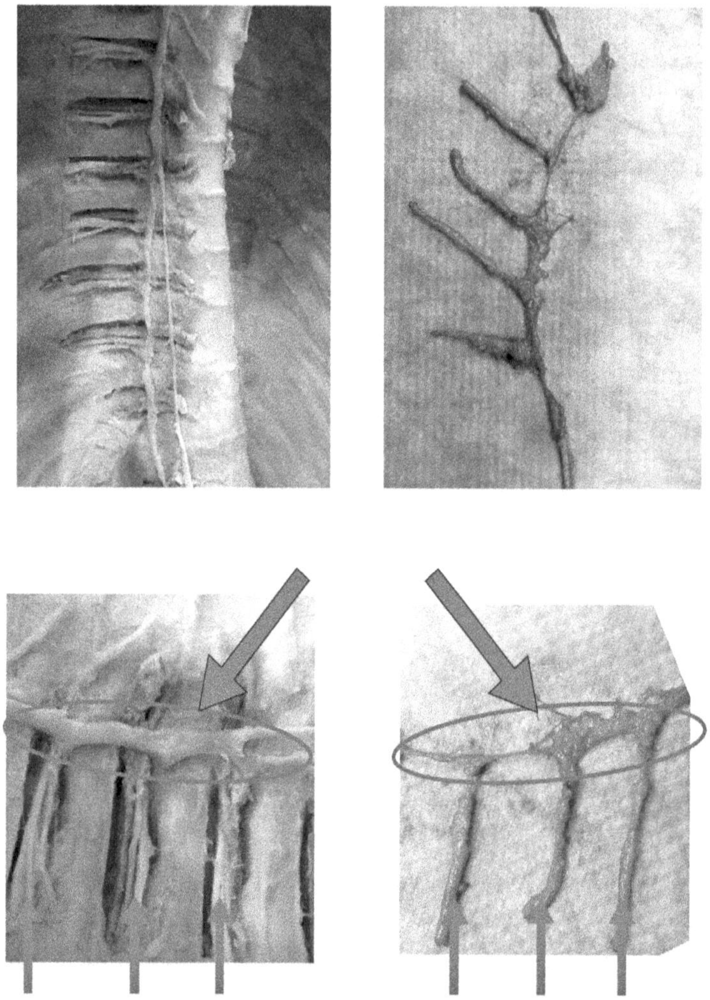

The sympathetic chain runs perpendicular to the spinal nerves under the ribs. The images on the left are from a plasticized human and on the right from a freshly obtained autopsy specimen. Small arrows show spinal nerves, large arrows sympathetic chain.

To convey what the ganglia of the autonomic nervous system do, think of how electricity is delivered to your home. From the generator plant and distribution center come thick, high voltage lines that transmit electricity along large towers. Outside your house is a utility pole that contains a transformer. From the utility pole much thinner, low voltage wires connect to your house.

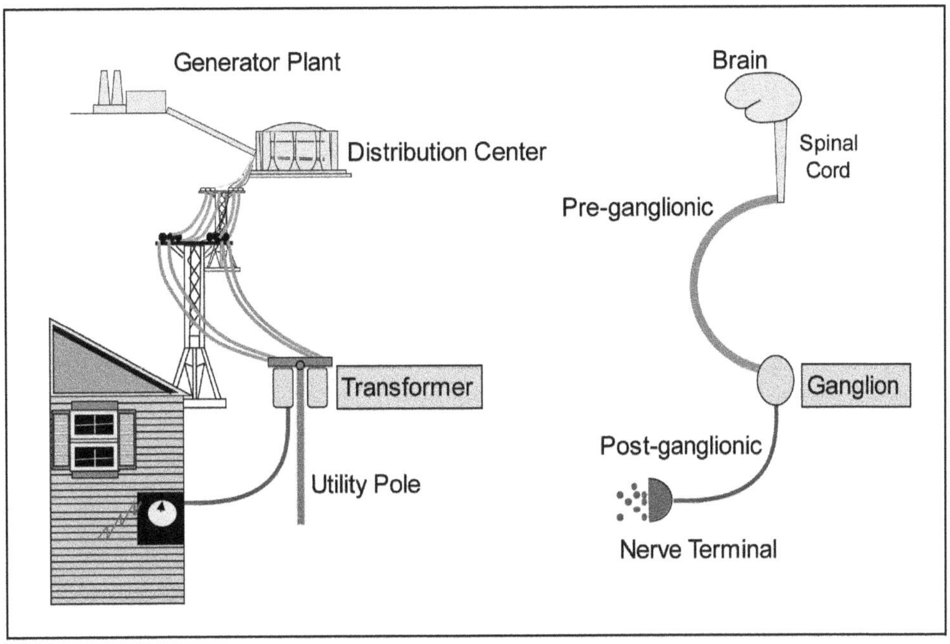

The ganglia act like transformer boxes on the utility pole outside your house.

The nerves from the spinal cord are called "pre-ganglionic." They are thick and conduct electricity quickly, because they have a myelin sheath. Myelin is a complex chemical consisting mainly of water, fat, and protein that appears white to the eye. The "white matter" of the brain is white because of myelin, and myelinated nerves look white. Electric signals are conducted more rapidly in myelinated than in non-myelinated nerves. The nerves from the ganglia to the target organs are "post-ganglionic." They are thin, slow conducting, and non-myelinated. They look gray.

In keeping with the idea that adrenaline is an emergency hormone that should be released rapidly, the cells of the adrenal gland that release adrenaline into the bloodstream receive myelinated nerve fibers, as if there were a direct wiring connection from the electrical distribution center to the terminal box.

The ANS has parts

About the turn of the 20th century, the English physiologist, John Newport Langley, proposed the existence of the "autonomic nervous system" (ANS). Langley invented this phrase.

He was referring to networks of nerves outside the central nervous system that are derived from ganglia. He described three components of the ANS— sympathetic, parasympathetic (a word he invented), and enteric. Sympathetic nerves are derived from the thoraco-lumbar spinal cord and parasympathetic nerves from the brainstem and sacral spinal cord, while enteric neurons are found within the walls of the gastrointestinal tract. The phrase, "sympathetic nervous system," goes back to ancient times—to the 2d century Greek physician, Galen.

Galen's ideas and teachings dominated medical thought and practice for 14 centuries. Galen taught that the body has "spirits"—animal, vital, and natural—and he viewed the nerves as conduits for delivering the animal spirits to body organs. The organs would then function in harmony with each other, in concert with each other—in "sympathy" with each other. No one ever has come up with evidence for the existence of the spirits; however, the idea that the sympathetic nervous system coordinates functions of body organs is essentially, ironically correct.

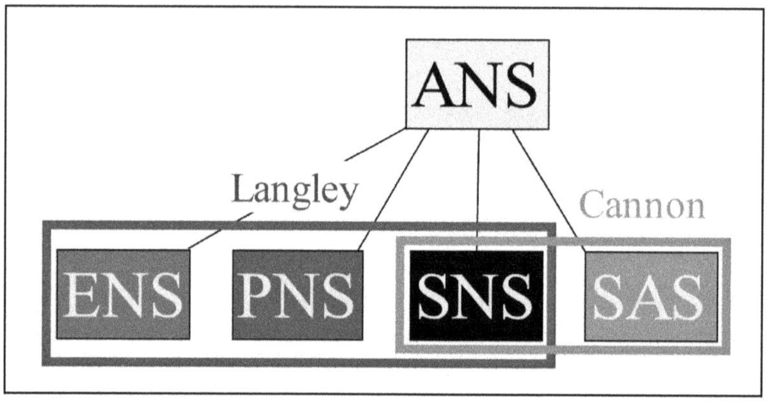

Langley's "autonomic nervous system" (ANS). ENS=enteric nervous system; PNS=parasympathetic nervous system; SNS=sympathetic nervous system.

Within several years after Langley formulated his idea of the ANS, the American physiologist, Walter B. Cannon, added what can be considered to be a fourth component of the ANS. I call it the sympathetic adrenergic system (SAS). This is the part of the autonomic nervous system where epinephrine (synonymous with adrenaline) is released from the inner part (medulla, from the Latin word for "marrow") of the adrenal gland. The SAS is a form of what would now be called a neuroendocrine system. The outer part of the adrenal gland, the cortex (from the Latin word for "bark," as in the bark of a tree) is the source of a variety of steroid hormones that are also very important in the body economy.

Cannon was the first to describe epinephrine release from the adrenal glands into the bloodstream during emotional distress. He drew blood from a cat exposed to a barking dog. This evoked release into the cat's blood of a substance that relaxed a strip of gut tissue. Exposure of the strip to blood from the adrenal veins produced the same relaxing effect, and tying off the adrenal veins eliminated the effect, indicating that distress released a substance from the adrenal glands into the bloodstream.

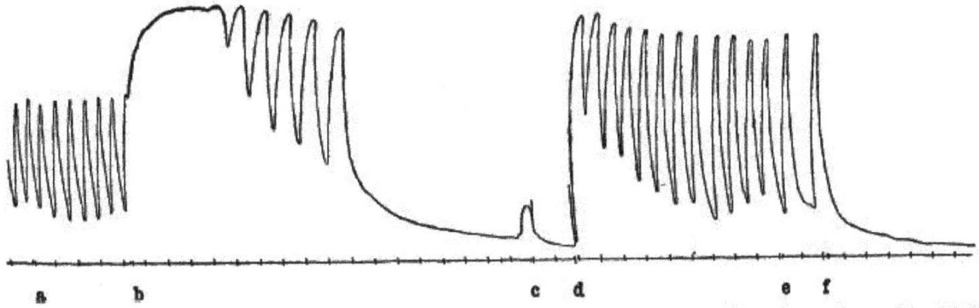

FIGURE 2.—About two fifths the original size. Alternatc application of excited blood (at *b* and *f*) and quiet blood (at *d*), from the same animal, to an intestinal strip initially beating in Ringer's solution. See text for further description.

Walter B. Cannon was the first to demonstrate epinephrine release from the adrenal gland during distress.

Cannon taught that the sympathetic nervous system and adrenal gland act as a functional unit in emergencies. This functional unit has been called the "sympathico-adrenal," "sympathoadrenomedullary," or "sympathoadrenal system."

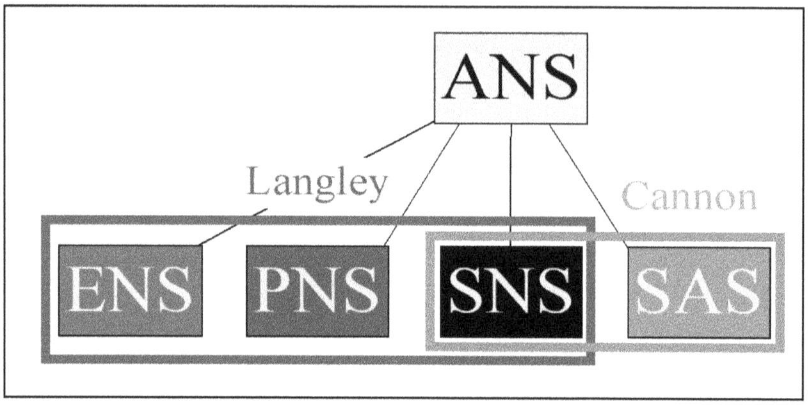

Cannon viewed the "sympathico-adrenal" system as a unitary emergency system. The sympathetic adrenergic system (SAS) was the first described neuroendocrine system.

According to Cannon, this system mediates bodily changes in "fight-or-flight" situations. ("Fight-or-flight" is a term he introduced.) He viewed the sympathoadrenal system as the key effector for maintaining "homeostasis" (a word he invented).

In the 1930s Sir Henry Dale (Nobel Prize, 1936) added what may be considered a fifth component of the autonomic nervous system, the sympathetic cholinergic system, or SCS.

The sympathetic cholinergic system is the main ANS component involved with sweating when you are exposed to environmental heat (thermoregulatory sweating).

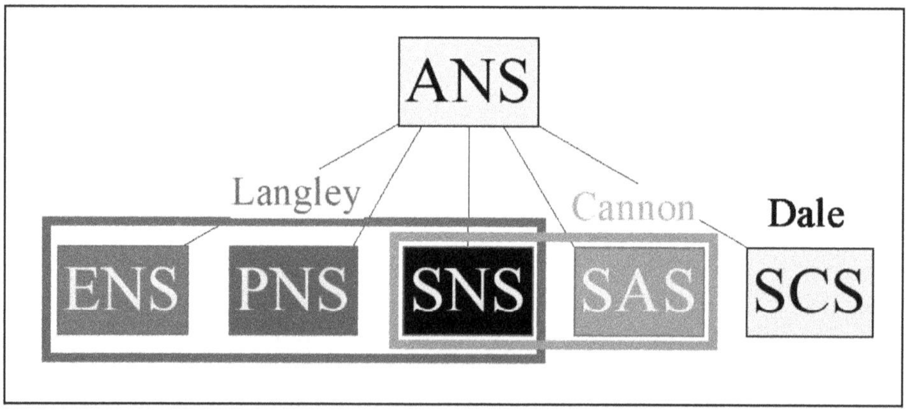

The ANS can be conceptualized in terms of having 5 components.

Organization of the ANS

This section is about how components of the autonomic nervous system are distributed in the body.

Parasympathetic nervous System (PNS)

You can think of the parasympathetic nervous system as regulating "vegetative" body functions—things you do privately or at night. The parasympathetic nervous system (PNS) in some ways acts like the opposite of an emergency system. Increased activity of this system is associated with "vegetative" behaviors, activities that increase rather than use up energy. Examples are sleeping, eating, salivating, and digesting.

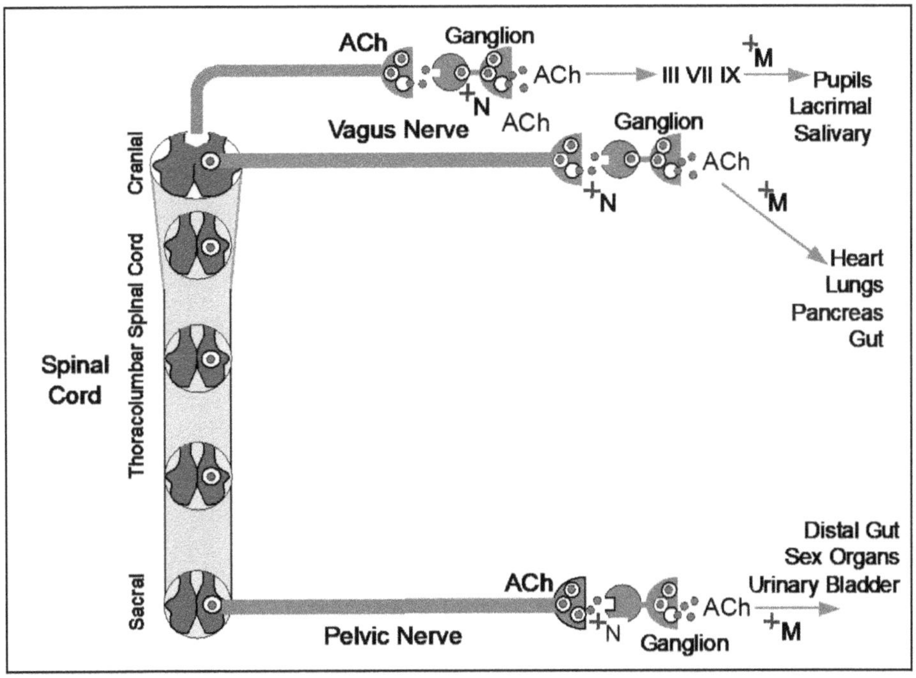

Overview of the organization of the parasympathetic nervous system.

The upper part of the parasympathetic nervous system consists of nerves that come from the brainstem. These nerves travel to many parts of your body, including the eyes, face, tongue, heart, and most of the gastrointestinal tract. Stimulation of the parasympathetic fibers in the head causes the pupils to constrict, the lacrimal glands to secrete tears, and the salivary glands to secrete watery saliva.

The parasympathetic fibers to the head are considered (somewhat irrationally, I would say) to be part of the peripheral nervous system, even though they travel in cranial nerves. This is because the parasympathetic nerves to the target structures are post-ganglionic. For instance, parasympathetic nerves supplying the sphincter muscle of the iris come from the ciliary ganglion, those supplying the lacrimal glands come from the sphenopalatine ganglion, and those supplying the salivary glands come from the submaxillary or otic ganglion. As for other ganglia that contain parasympathetic nerves, these ganglia are located near or in the innervated structures.

The vagus nerve, which is the tenth cranial nerve (cranial nerve X), comes from the lower brainstem. The vagus contains most of the parasympathetic nerves in the body.

"Vagus" comes from the Latin word for wandering. As the name suggests, the vagus goes to several places inside the chest, abdomen, and pelvis, and it supplies the heart, lungs, and most of the gastrointestinal tract.

Stimulation of the vagus nerve decreases the heart rate, increases smooth muscle tone and mucus secretion in the airways, and increases secretion of stomach acid and digestive hormones such as insulin. Vagal stimulation also decreases the force of cardiac contraction (in contrast with an older teaching that there is no effect).

There are ganglia within the heart muscle (intrinsic ganglia), just as there are intrinsic ganglia in the wall of the gastrointestinal tract. It is possible that intrinsic ganglia are phylogenetically ancient and were superseded during the course of evolution by hormones and autonomic nerve networks.

Most of the nerve fibers in the vagus actually are afferents, meaning that carry signals to the brain, rather than carrying signals from the brain. As you will learn later, a scientifically and clinically important source of afferent signals to the brain is distortion receptors (baroreceptors) in the walls of the heart, large arteries, and pulmonary veins.

The lower part of the parasympathetic nervous system consists of nerves from the bottom level of the spinal cord, the sacral spinal cord. These nerves travel to the lower gastrointestinal tract, urinary bladder, and genital organs.

Sacral parasympathetic stimulation increases peristalsis in the colon and contraction of the rectum while relaxing the anal sphincter, so that defecation occurs. Such stimulation also increases peristalsis in the ureters and activates the detrusor muscle of the urinary bladder while relaxing the urethral sphincter, so that urination occurs. Parasympathetic stimulation augments filling of the corpora cavernosum and corpus spongiosum of the penis with blood and thereby promotes penile erection.

Interference with sacral parasympathetic outflows manifests with constipation, urinary retention, and erectile dysfunction in men.

Parasympathetic nervous system failure produces many symptoms, including dry mouth, constipation, urinary problems, decreased tear production, and (in men) inability to have an erection.

Sympathetic noradrenergic system (SNS)

You can think of the sympathetic noradrenergic system (SNS) as the part of the autonomic nervous system involved with processes that happen during the day or out in the open.

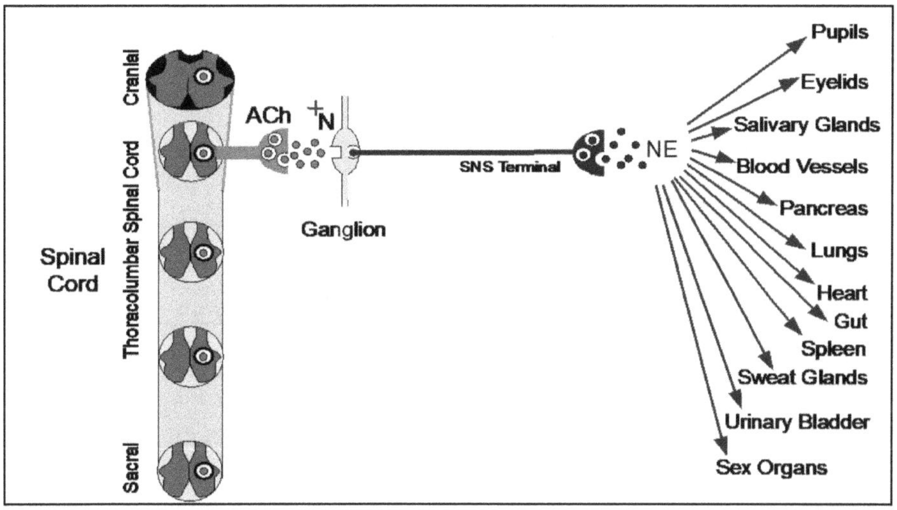

Overview of the organization of the sympathetic noradrenergic system (SNS).

The nerves of the SNS come from the spinal cord at the levels of the chest and upper abdomen (thoracolumbar spinal cord). The sympathetic nerves to most organs are post-ganglionic, coming from cell bodies in the ganglia, the clusters of nerve cells like a transformer on the utility pole that supplies the electricity to your house.

Probably the most prominent effect of stimulation of the SNS is constriction of blood vessels—especially of arterioles, the tiny arteries that are the main determinant of total peripheral resistance to blood flow in the body. Decreased blood flow to the skin causes pallor. Blood flow is also decreased to the gut, skeletal muscles, and kidneys, and so the blood pressure increases. Blood flow to vital organs—the heart, lungs, and brain—is generally preserved during SNS stimulation.

Sympathetic adrenergic system (SAS)

The sympathetic adrenergic system (abbreviated as SAS), or adrenomedullary hormonal system, is the part of the autonomic nervous system for which epinephrine (adrenaline) is the main chemical messenger.

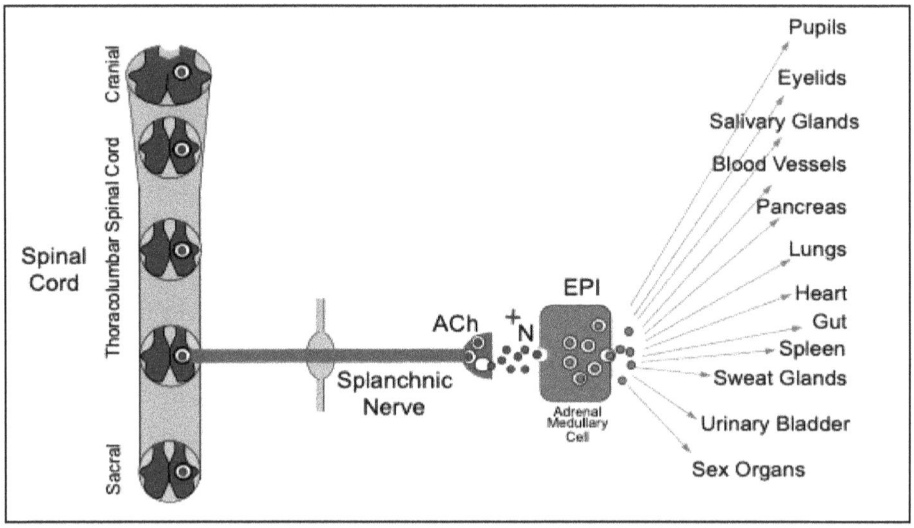

Overview of the organization of the sympathetic adrenergic system (SAS).

The location of the adrenal glands explains the origins of the word, adrenaline, from the Latin words for "near the kidney," and of the word, epinephrine, from the Greek words for "on the kidney."

The SAS regulates "emergency" processes such as in distress. Any threat to survival increases adrenaline levels. The SAS plays a major role in responses to perceived or anticipated threats to overall homeostasis, such as lack of essential fuels (glucose and oxygen), inadequate blood flow to vital organs, and hostile encounters.

In the SAS, the connection from the spinal cord to the adrenal medullary cells is direct, and so the adrenal medulla receives rapidly conducting, myelinated fibers. This fits with the teleologic notion of adrenaline being released with the goal to maintain homeostasis in sudden emergencies. We will return later to the concepts of teleology and homeostasis. Epinephrine is secreted into the bloodstream and distributed widely in the body, so it is a hormone. A major determinant of its release is myelinated nerve fibers passing through the splanchnic ganglia. This means that the SAS is also a neuro- hormonal, or neuroendocrine, system.

SAS activation potently increases blood flow to skeletal muscle. Probably the systemic cardiovascular effect of adrenaline that occurs at the lowest concentration is a fall in skeletal muscle vascular resistance. At higher concentrations, epinephrine produces well known stimulation of the heart, increasing both the rate and force of contraction, and constricts blood vessels by stimulating alpha-adrenoceptors. Adrenaline also causes pallor, relaxes the gut, increases sweating, increases blood glucose levels, decreases serum potassium levels, and increases the core temperature.

Sympathetic cholinergic system (SCS)

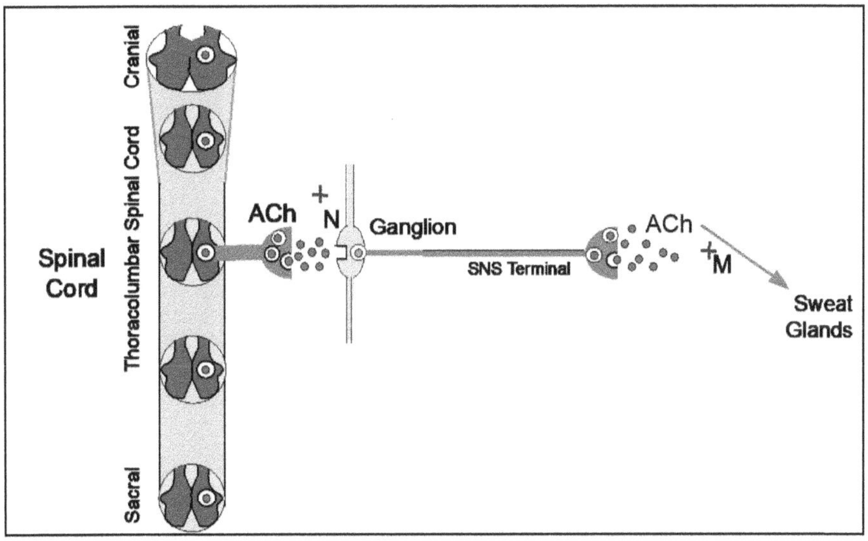

The sympathetic cholinergic system consists mainly of non-myelinated post-ganglionic nerves that supply sweat glands.

The sympathetic cholinergic system (SCS) mediates sweating—especially thermoregulatory sweating, when you perspire upon exposure to heat. The SCS also participates in gustatory sweating when you sweat on your forehead after you eat spicy foods, and in emotional sweating when your palms and armpits sweat during distress.

Eccrine sweat glands (from the Greek word for "secrete"), which are the major sweat glands in the human body, occur at highest density in the palms, soles, and head. They secrete watery, salty, odorless sweat and are the main mediators of thermoregulatory sweating. Eccrine sweat glands receive prominent sympathetic cholinergic fibers, which are long, post- ganglionic, and non-myelinated.

Apocrine sweat glands (from the Greek words for "separate" and "away"), release sweat near hair follicles and occur at high density in the armpits, groin, and peri-anal area, as well as in the nostrils, ear canals, and areolae of the nipples. Apocrine sweat glands secrete oily, opaque sweat; its characteristic odor results from metabolic breakdown by local bacteria. This is the type of sweating associated with severe exercise and strong emotions.

Enteric nervous system (ENS)

The intrinsic neurons of the ENS (ganglion cells) migrate from the neural crest during fetal development. The ganglion cells are required for movement of intestinal contents.

The ganglion cells of the ENS are in two plexuses, Auerbach's myenteric plexus, in the layer of outer longitudinal muscle, and Meissner's submucosal plexus. Auerbach's myenteric plexus receives parasympathetic post-ganglioic innervation. There also is SNS innervation of the gut, and as noted above EPI potently inhibits gastrointestinal movements. This means that autonomic regulation of the gut involves 4 of the components of the ANS.

As you will learn in more detail later, in Hirschsprung's disease this migration is incomplete, and the affected segment of the colon that lacks the ganglion cells cannot relax and move stool through the colon. Hirschsprung's disease therefore manifests clinically with failure of the newborn to pass meconium or stool.

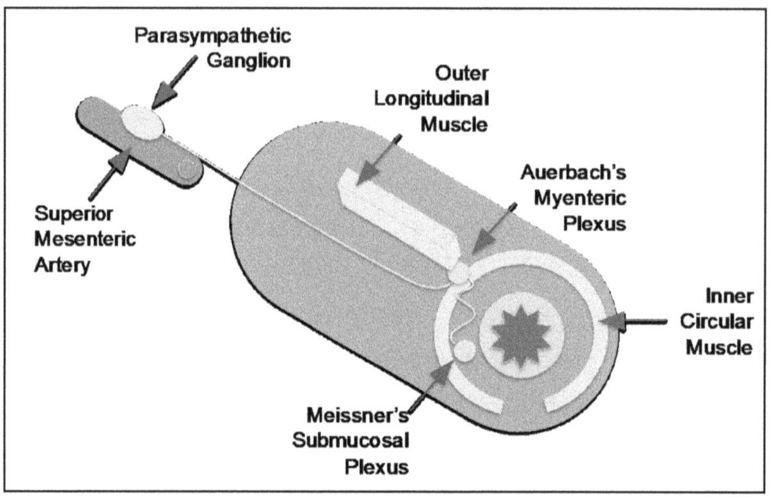

Overview of the organization of the enteric nervous system (ENS).

Interactions among ANS components

Activation of a particular component of the ANS can lead to effects on other components. This is an important principle of autonomic medicine.

For instance, the sympathetic noradrenergic system (SNS) and the parasympathetic nervous system (PNS) seem to antagonize each other. When sympathetic nerves in the heart are stimulated, the heart rate speeds up, and the heart beats more forcefully, whereas when parasympathetic nerves in the heart are stimulated, the heart rate slows down, and the heart beats less forcefully.

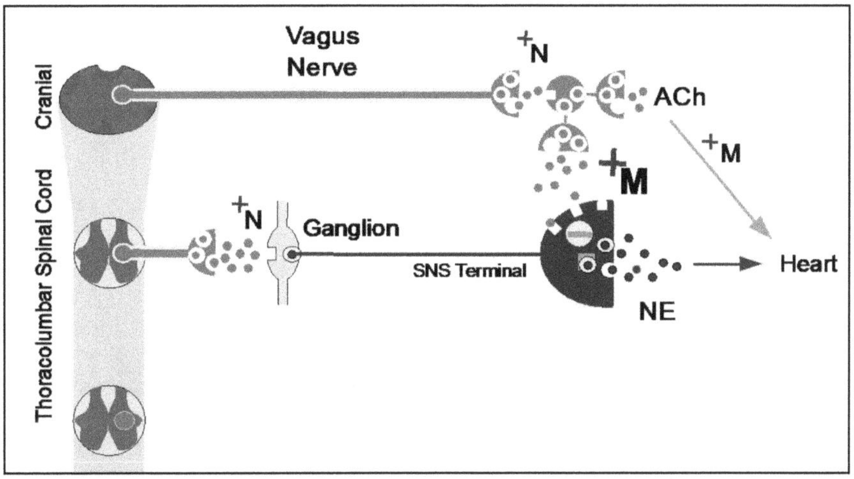

Vagal activation stimulates muscarinic acetylcholine receptors (+M) on SNS terminals in the heart, inhibiting NE release.

Parasympathetic cardiovagal stimulation decreases the rate and force of cardiac contraction directly as well as indirectly, by inhibiting release of the chemical messenger norepinephrine (NE) from sympathetic post-ganglionic nerves.

Autonomic innervation of the pupils

Autonomic influences on pupillary diameter occur via three systems—the PNS, via the oculomotor nerve, the SNS, via the ophthalmic nerve, and the SAS, via circulating epinephrine (EPI).

Pupil constriction evoked by PNS stimulation is mediated by acetylcholine acting at muscarinic receptors on iris sphincter muscle cells. The nerve fibers travel in the oculomotor nerve, which is the third cranial nerve, via the ciliary ganglion. The sphincter muscle cells are arranged circularly in the iris, and so when they contract the pupils get smaller.

The SNS innervation of the pupils is derived from pre-ganglionic neurons in the thoracic spinal cord. The nerve fibers synapse in the superior cervical ganglion in the neck and travel with the ophthalmic nerve, which is part of the fifth cranial nerve (the trigeminal nerve).

The pupillary dilation evoked by SNS stimulation is mediated by NE acting at alpha-1 adrenoceptors on iris dilator muscle cells. The iris dilator cells are arranged radially (like spokes on a bicycle wheel) in the iris, and so when they contract the pupils get larger.

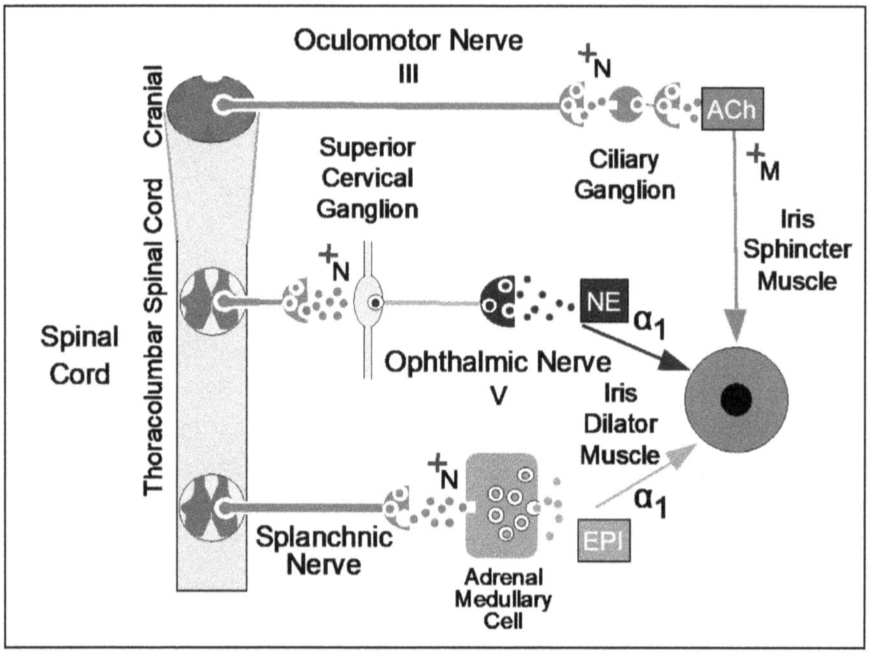

Three components of the ANS affect pupillary diameter.

Activation of the sympathetic adrenergic system (SAS), such as during distress, causes release of EPI into the bloodstream. EPI also acts at the alpha-1 adrenoceptors on iris dilator muscle cells and dilates the pupils. SAS activation probably explains the pupillary dilation that occurs when people faint.

SNS vs. PNS: not always a yin-yang

There are situations where the SNS and PNS do not usually antagonize each other. After eating a meal, increased activity of the PNS aids digestion, by increasing gut motions and augmenting secretion of hormones such as insulin. Meanwhile, patterned activation of the SNS tightens blood vessels in other organs shunts blood toward the gut. Possibly because of increased levels of glucose in the bloodstream, activity of the sympathetic adrenergic system (SAS) tends to decrease.

Fainting typically involves a particular pattern of changes in activities of components of the autonomic nervous system. When people faint, vagal outflow is activated, producing changes such as nausea and retching. Activity of the SNS often is decreased, resulting in a fall in blood pressure. The SAS is stimulated markedly, and this shunts blood toward the skeletal muscle. High circulating epinephrine levels are probably responsible for constriction of blood vessels in the skin, resulting in pallor, and for dilation of the pupils. Finally, when people faint they typically have increased sweating. This might reflect increased activity of the sympathetic cholinergic system but could result from effects of high circulating EPI levels.

Summary of the organization of the ANS

Let's review the information so far about the ANS. It can be a bit confusing, because of the different "nervous systems" involved.

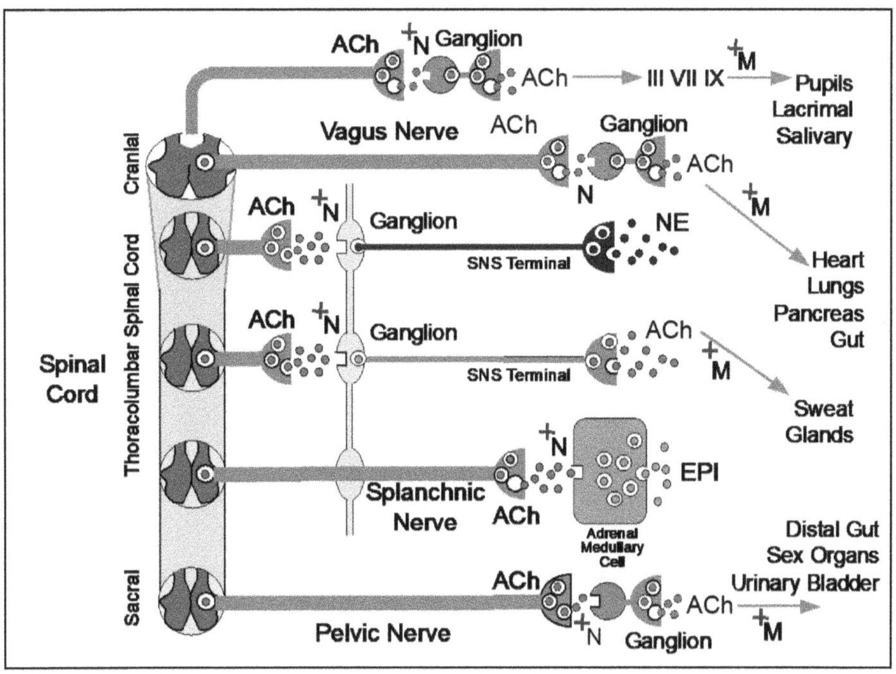

Summary of the organization of the autonomic nervous system.

You have a central nervous system (your brain and spinal cord) and a peripheral nervous system (the rest of your nerves). The latter has two divisions, the somatic nervous system and the autonomic nervous system (ANS). The somatic nervous system is concerned with the "outer world," and the nerves in this system travel to skeletal muscle.

Your ANS is concerned with the "inner world" within the body, and it usually works automatically, so that you can think of the autonomic nervous system as the "automatic nervous system."

The control signals of the ANS travel indirectly from your central nervous system through ganglia (clusters of nerve cells) to smooth muscle, found in areas like your blood vessels, heart, and glands throughout the body. Nerves coming to the ganglia from the spinal cord are pre-ganglionic, and nerves coming from the ganglia are post-ganglionic. Some nerves, such as those to the adrenal glands, pass through the ganglia without relaying within the ganglia, so that there is a direct connection from the central nervous system to the target organs.

You have also learned that there are several components of the ANS. Two of the main components are the sympathetic nervous system (SNS) and the parasympathetic nervous system (PNS).

The adrenal glands, located near the tops of the kidneys, are the source of the hormone epinephrine (EPI, adrenaline). The combination of the adrenal medulla with the sympathetic nervous system has been called the "sympathoadrenal system," which has been thought to function as a unit in emergencies such as "fight-or-flight" situations. Sometimes components of the ANS work together, and sometimes they antagonize each other. The interactions of ANS components often occur in characteristic patterns.

Finally, you have learned about the distribution of autonomic nerves in the body. Parasympathetic nerves come from the brainstem and sacral spinal cord, and sympathetic nerves (noradrenergic, adrenergic, and cholinergic) come from the thoracolumbar spinal cord. Parasympathetic nerves have long, myelinated pre-ganglionic and short, non-myelinated post-ganglionic fibers. Sympathetic nerves have short, myelinated pre-ganglionic fibers and long, non-myelinated post-ganglionic fibers. Sympathetic adrenergic nerves supplying the adrenal medulla are myelinated, but instead of post-ganglionic nerves the adrenal medullary cells secrete EPI into the bloodstream.

Now that you've learned about the components of the ANS and its anatomic organization in the body, it is time to cover how the ANS works. This is crucial for understanding what goes wrong in dysautonomias, how to diagnose them, and how to treat them.

HOW DOES THE ANS WORK?

The autonomic nervous system works by releasing chemicals inside the body.

Some understanding of clinical neurochemistry is required to grasp concepts about mechanisms, testing, and treatment of autonomic disorders.

In general, chemical messaging in the ANS is by neurotransmitters, hormones, and autocrine-paracrine substances.

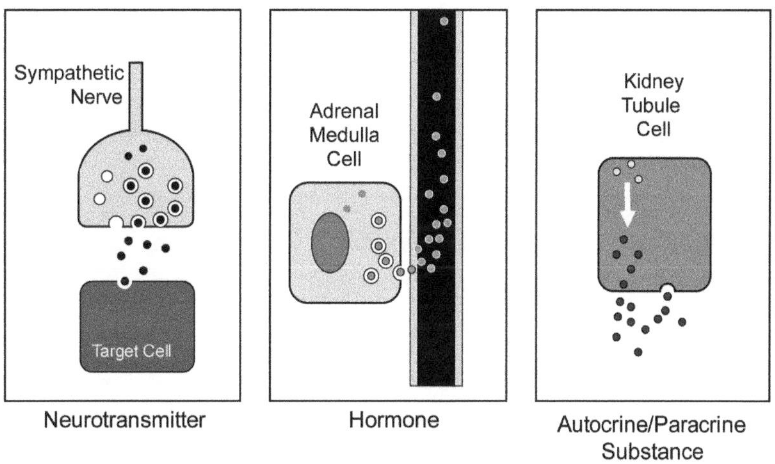

Three types of chemical messaging in the ANS: Neurotransmitters, hormones, and autocrine-paracrine substances.

Chemical Messengers of the ANS

Neurotransmitters

Neurotransmitters are chemical messengers that are released from nerves and produce effects at nearby target cells within the organ.

Neurotransmitters released from nerves act locally and are inactivated locally. Only a small fraction of released neurotransmitters make their way to the bloodstream unchanged. This makes it complex or impossible to monitor release of neurotransmitters by measuring levels in the plasma.

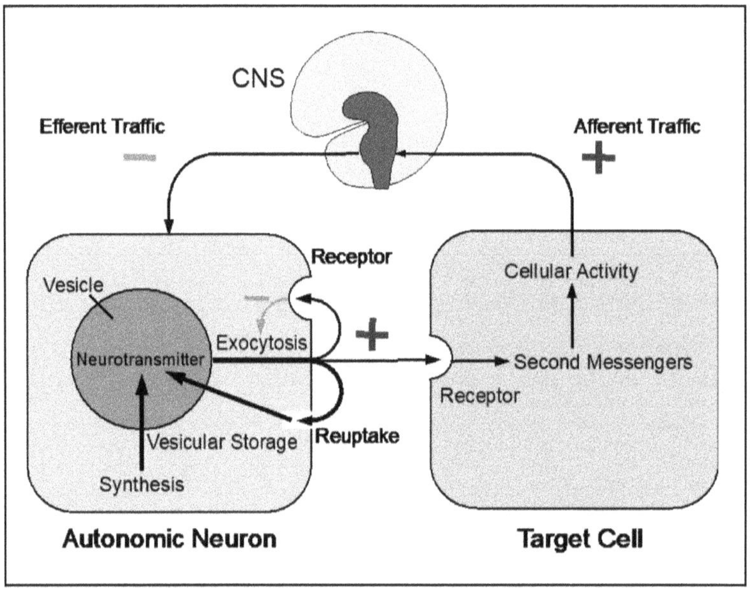

Some common themes in chemical messaging by neurotransmitter systems in the ANS.

Key steps in the functioning of the neurotransmitter systems of the ANS are:

1. Production (synthesis) of the chemical messengers.
2. Storage of the messengers in bubble-like vesicles by vesicular uptake.
3. Release of the chemical messengers by fusion of the vesicles with the membrane surface, followed by formation of holes at the vesicle-membrane junction (poration) and release of the contents of the vesicles into the interstitial fluid (exocytosis).
4. Vesicular recycling by the vesicles coming off the membrane surface and going back to the cytoplasm (endocytosis). Another form of recycling is via neuronal reuptake of released neurotransmitters, mediated by specific cell membrane transporters.
5. Metabolism of the chemical messengers.

6. Binding of the chemical messengers to receptors on the target cells. The neurotransmitter may bind to receptors on the nerve terminal (autoreceptors), modulating the amount of release for a given amount of nerve traffic.
7. Second messengers that relate receptor occupation to cellular activation or inhibition.
8. Afferent nerve traffic to the brain (especially to the nucleus of the solitary tract (NTS) in the back of the lowest part of the brainstem, the medulla.
9. Complex integration in the brain in the "central autonomic network."
10. Efferent nerve traffic from the brain down the spinal cord to neurons that project to the ganglia.

All these steps are tightly coordinated. One key way this coordination occurs is by negative feedback regulation. We'll be returning to this many times later on. In the concept diagram, a process that is stimulatory is indicated by a (+) sign, and a process that is inhibitory is indicated by a (-) sign.

Hormones

Hormones are released directly into the bloodstream and are delivered to most body organs. One of the most famous hormones—and the first to be identified—epinephrine (EPI, adrenaline), which is released by the adrenal gland.

The sympathetic adrenergic system (SAS) can be viewed as a neuroendocrine system, because nervous stimulation leads to release of the hormone, EPI. One may reasonably argue that EPI was the first neuroendocrine substance to be identified. Other major neuroendocrine hormones of the body include cortisol, insulin, and gastrin. It may be reasonable to conceptualize that neuroendocrine systems expand the meaning of the term, autonomic.

Another extension of the concept of autonomic relates to the immune system. A large family of proteins called cytokines are released from cells of the immune system. Cytokines play key roles in immunity and bodily responses to infection, inflammation, trauma, sepsis, and cancer. Neuroimmunology is a rapidly evolving field that focuses on interactions between the nervous system (including the ANS) and immune functions.

We will be returning to interactions among autonomic, neuroendocrine, and immune/inflammatory systems and the integration of all three by the central autonomic network near the end of this book, in the section "Ideas for the future."

Autocrine-paracrine substances

Besides neurotransmitters and hormones, a third type of chemical messenger—probably the oldest in evolutionary terms—involves a class of chemicals called autocrine/paracrine substances. These chemicals are made in, released from, and act on the same or nearby target cells.

Unlike hormones and neurotransmitters, which are stored at particular sites within cells and are released from the storage sites in response to nerve traffic, autocrine/paracrine substances are released as soon as they are made within the cells.

Two cholinergic systems

The ANS has two types of cholinergic neurotransmitter systems, in which acetylcholine (ACh) is the main chemical messenger. The first and most well-known is the parasympathetic nervous system (PNS), which includes the vagus nerve. The second is the sympathetic cholinergic system (SCS), in which post-ganglionic sympathetic nerves supply the sweat glands.

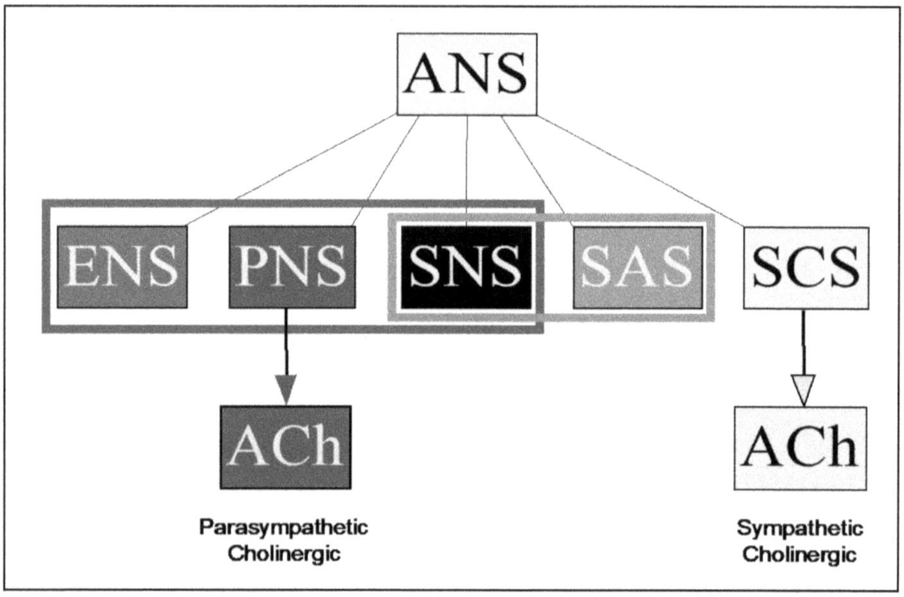

The ANS includes 2 components where acetylcholine (ACh) is the neurotransmitter, the parasympathetic nervous system (PNS) and the sympathetic cholinergic system (SCS).

This means that blockade of cholinergic receptors decreases sweating, whereas failure of the PNS does not. On the other hand, failure of the PNS, which includes not only the vagus nerve but also nerves supplying the salivary glands, lacrimal glands, and pupils, results in dry mouth, dry eyes, and pupillary dilation, whereas SCS failure does not.

Three routes to sympathy

Since acetylcholine is the neurotransmitter of the sympathetic cholinergic system (SCS), one can conceptualize three neurotransmitters of the sympathetic nervous system—norepinephrine (NE), epinephrine (EPI), and acetylcholine (ACh).

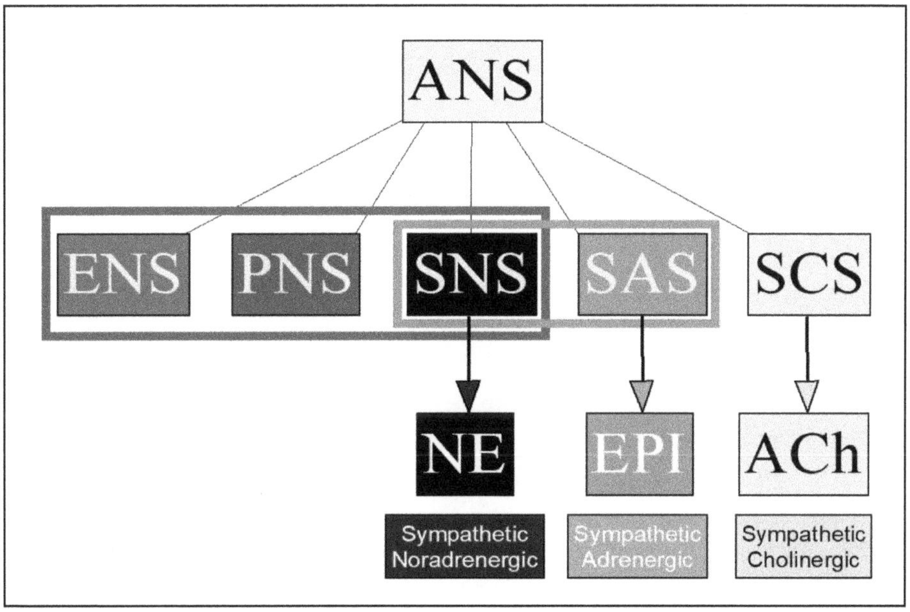

The sympathetic nervous system has 3 components with different chemical messengers. Norepinephrine (NE) is the neurotransmitter of the sympathetic noradrenergic system (SNS), epinephrine (EPI) is the hormone of the sympathetic adrenergic system (SAS), and acetylcholine (ACh) is the neurotransmitter of the sympathetic cholinergic system (SCS).

There is no single neurotransmitter of the enteric nervous system (ENS). There are many, and they interact in a highly complex manner. I think of the ENS as a conglomerate of intrinsic neurons, neurotransmitter systems, hormones, and autocrine-paracrine systems.

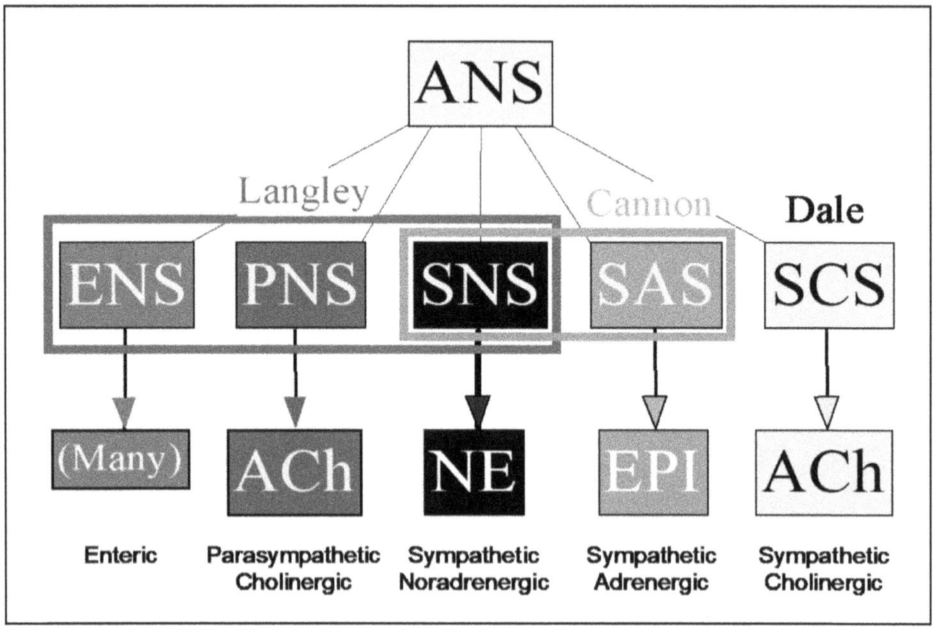

Overview of chemical messengers of the ANS. Langley's ANS includes the enteric nervous system (ENS), parasympathetic nervous system (PNS), and sympathetic nervous system. Cannon conceptualized a unitary sympathoadrenal system. The sympathetic noradrenergic system (SNS) uses norepinephrine (NE) as the neurotransmitter, and the sympathetic adrenergic system (SAS) uses the hormone epinephrine (EPI) as the chemical messenger. The ENS entails many chemical messengers. Dale described sweating mediated by the sympathetic cholinergic system (SCS).

The human body uses three catecholamines as chemical messengers. In addition to NE and EPI there is dopamine (DA). In the brain NE and DA are major neurotransmitters. Outside the brain, DA acts as an autocrine-paracrine substance. This means that the three catecholamines of the body, NE, EPI, and DA, exemplify three types of chemical messenger systems.

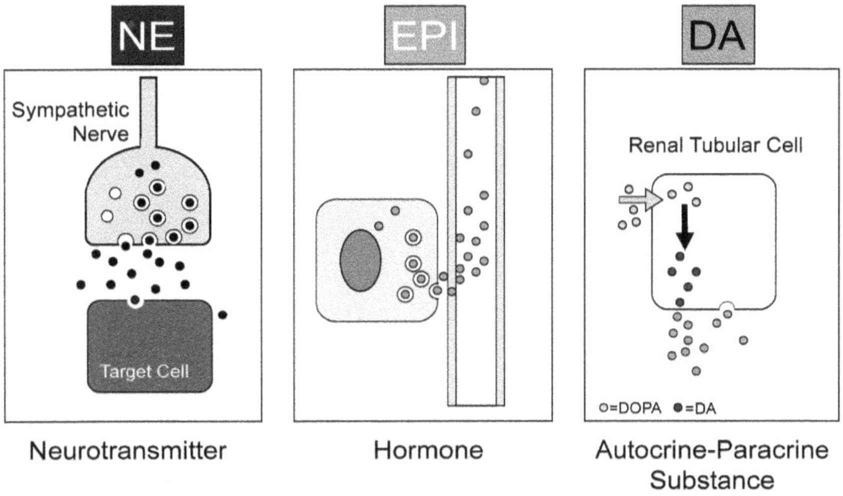

NE is the neurotransmitter of the SNS, EPI is the hormone of the SAS, and DA is the autocrine-paracrine substance of the renal DOPA-dopamine system.

Of several autocrine/paracrine substances in the body, one involves the catecholamine, dopamine. In proximal tubular cells of the kidneys, DOPA is converted to DA by the enzyme L-aromatic-amino-acid decarboxylase (LAAAD). DA released from the cells act on receptors of the same or nearby cells. This increases excretion of sodium and water.

Catechols look like Cats

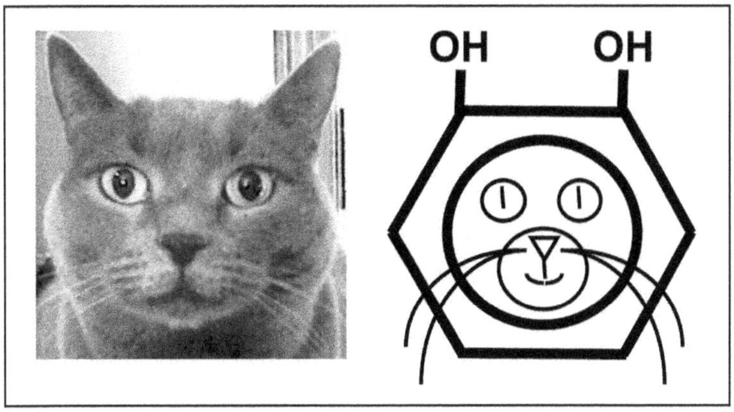

The chemical, catechol, has a particular structure, consisting of a hexagon of carbon atoms with hydroxyl (OH) groups attached to adjacent points of the hexagon. The hexagonal ring is the face. The two hydroxyl groups are the pointy ears.

The catecholamines of the body—norepinephrine, adrenaline, and dopamine—are catechols.

Catechol itself does not exist in the human body, but chemicals that contain catechol as part of their molecular structure are called catechols.

A catecholamine is a catechol that has a hydrocarbon tail ending in an amine (ammonia) group. Think of the cat in its litter box, with the ammonia coming off the tail end producing a smell like urine.

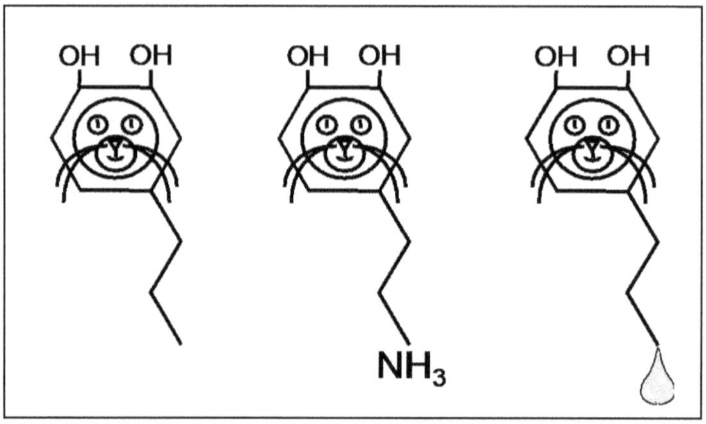

A catecholamine is like the entire cat from head to tail—in its litterbox.

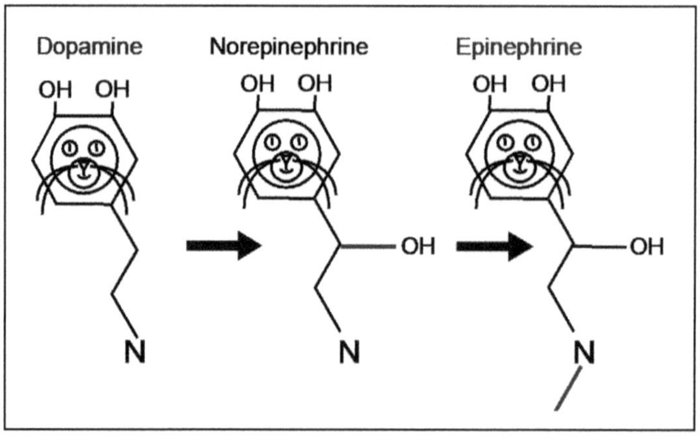

Dopamine is converted to norepinephrine, and norepinephrine is converted to epinephrine.

The body's catecholamines come from DOPA (technically 3,4-dihydroxy-phenylalanine), which is an amino acid, and DOPA comes from tyrosine, which is also an amino acid. Tyrosine is an amino acid that is not a catechol; DOPA is a catechol but is not a catecholamine.

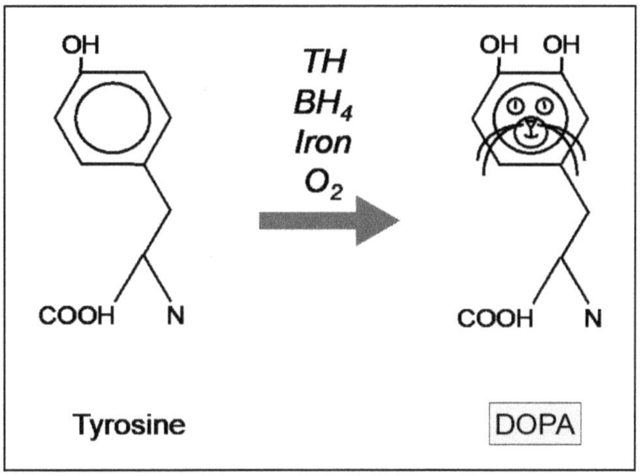

DOPA, the precursor of the catecholamines, is produced by the action of tyrosine hydroxylase (TH) on the non-catechol amino acid tyrosine. Tetrahydrobiopterin (BH4) is a required cofactor for TH.

Tyrosine is converted to DOPA by the actions of an enzyme (a protein that speeds up a particular chemical process). The enzyme that speeds up the conversion of tyrosine to DOPA is tyrosine hydroxylase (TH). For TH to work requires oxygen, iron, and tetrahydrobiopterin, abbreviated BH4.

The next station on the catecholamine assembly line is the conversion of DOPA to DA, the grandfather in the catecholamine family. This step takes place in many types of cells and not just in cells that possess the rest of the machinery to store and recycle catecholamines. To make DA from DOPA requires the enzyme,

L-aromatic amino-acid decarboxylase (LAAAD, sometimes called DOPA decarboxylase, or DDC), and the co-factor pyridoxal phosphate, which is vitamin B6. (Incidentally, the word "vitamin" comes from "vital amine," even though some vitamins, such as vitamin B6, are not amines at all.)

DOPA is a neutral amino acid, and it is taken up by all types of cells in the body, because all cells express a neutral amino acid transporter. Many cell types, such as kidney and liver cells, contain abundant LAAAD, and in several organs DA is made from the DOPA after uptake of the DOPA from the bloodstream.

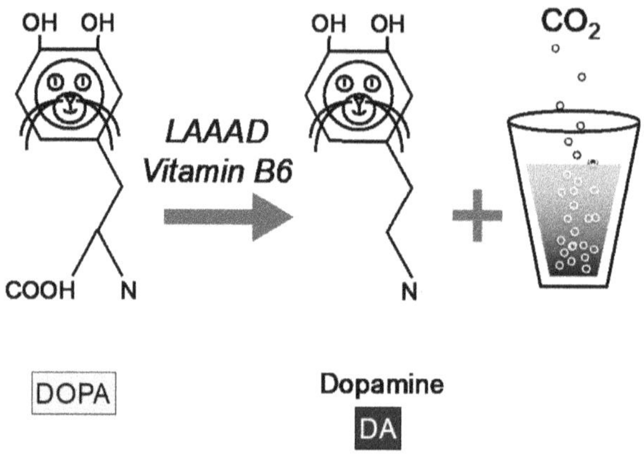

Dopamine is produced by the action of L-aromatic-amino-acid decarboxylase (LAAAD) on DOPA. Pyridoxal phosphate (vitamin B6) is a required cofactor for LAAAD.

The conversion of DOPA to DA involves cleaving off carbon dioxide from the molecule of DOPA. If this chemical reaction were carried out in a glass of water, the generated carbon dioxide gas would bubble up to the surface, like the effervescence in seltzer. Maybe this will help you remember that by this reaction DOPA turns into a cat-a-COLA-mean. (Actually, because of the rapid oxidation of dopamine in solution to form a tan breakdown product, it would be more accurate to think about the reaction generating ginger ale—but then there wouldn't be any pun with cola soda.)

Vesicular uptake and storage

Dopamine (DA) is made from DOPA in the cytoplasm ("cell juice") of neurons and cells that make catecholamines. For DA to be converted to norepinephrine (NE), however, DA must be taken up into tiny bubble-like structures called vesicles within the neurons or cells. All the chemical messengers of the autonomic nervous system, including NE, EPI, DA, and ACh, are stored in vesicles.

Unlike DA and ACh, which are produced in the cytoplasm and then actively pumped into the vesicles, NE is produced within the vesicles. This is because dopamine-beta-hydroxylase DBH), he enzyme that converts DA to NE, is localized to the vesicles in noradrenergic neurons and in cells of the adrenal medulla. In order to synthesize NE, DA must be taken up into the vesicles. In sympathetic noradrenergic nerves, adrenomedullary cells, and noradrenergic neurons in the brain, a transporter called the type 2 vesicular monoamine transporter (VMAT2) mediates the uptake of dopamine into the vesicles.

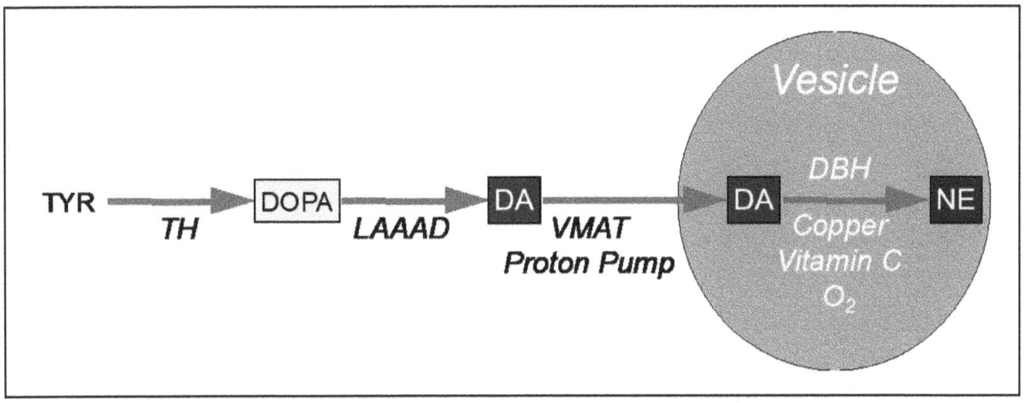

Norepinephrine (NE) is produced in vesicles after uptake of dopamine (DA) from the cytoplasm via the vesicular monoamine transporter (VMAT). Dopamine-beta-hydroxylase (DBH) is localized to the vesicles in NE-producing cells.

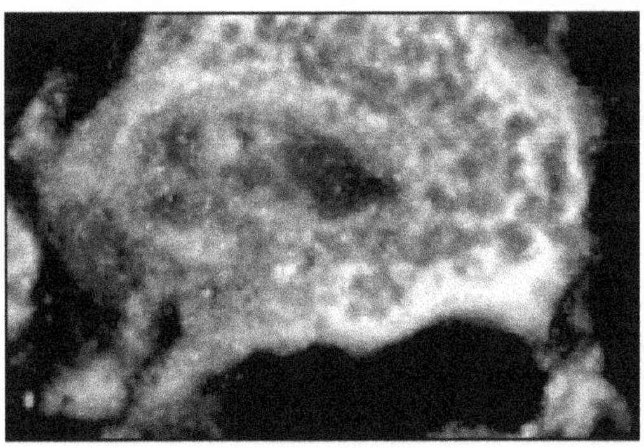

A noradrenergic cell in a human sympathetic ganglion. Dopamine-beta-hydroxylase (DBH) dots are numerous.

In the photomicrograph the DBH-containing vesicles seem to be arranged in clusters (the DBH-containing particles are too large to be vesicles themselves).

Vesicular uptake not only is a mechanism for packaging chemical messengers but also for detoxifying potentially toxic compounds that are in the cytoplasm. Vitamin C (ascorbic acid) is required for the transfer of electrons when DBH acts on vesicular DA.

DBH is a copper enzyme. DBH contains—and its activity absolutely depends on—copper. We will return to the importance of DBH being a copper enzyme later in the description of the pediatric disorder Menkes disease.

Vesicular uptake is an energy requiring process that uses adenosine triphosphate (ATP) for pumping protons into the vesicles by a proton pump. This makes the inside of the vesicles acidic. As the protons leak passively out of the vesicle, DA enters the vesicle via the VMAT.

Mitochondria in cells are the main source of ATP. Because vesicular uptake is an energy-requiring process, almost any problem that impedes mitochondrial functions can lead to decreased vesicular uptake of cytoplasmic catecholamines. Vesicular contents leak passively and continuously into the cytoplasm. Therefore, any cellular "energy crisis" in sympathetic noradrenergic neurons will lead to depletion of the neurotransmitter.

Stress vitamins

Production of NE and EPI requires at least two vitamins. The conversion of DOPA to DA depends on the availability of pyridoxal phosphate, which is vitamin B6.
The conversion of DA to NE requires ascorbic acid, which is vitamin C.

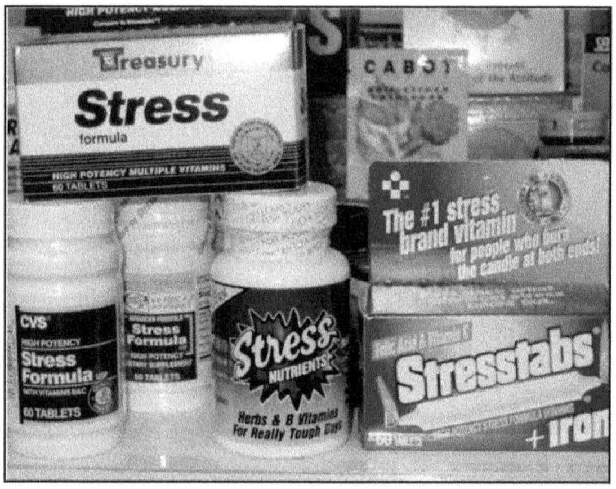

"Stress" formulas contain vitamin B6 and vitamin C. Both are required for norepinephrine and epinephrine synthesis.

"Stress" formulas contain vitamin B6 and vitamin C. Both are required for norepinephrine and epinephrine synthesis.

In my office I have a large "stress collection" consisting of items sold to alleviate stress. (A section later deals with the meaning of stress as a scientific idea.) As near as I can tell, all stress formulas contain vitamins B6 and C.

The adrenal bon-bon

EPI is NE with a methyl group added to the amine group at the end of the hydrocarbon tail in the NE molecule. S-adenosyl methionine (SAMe) is the source of the methyl group. The enzyme phenylethanolamine-N-methyltransferase (PNMT) catalyzes the transfer of the methyl group from SAMe to the amine group in NE.

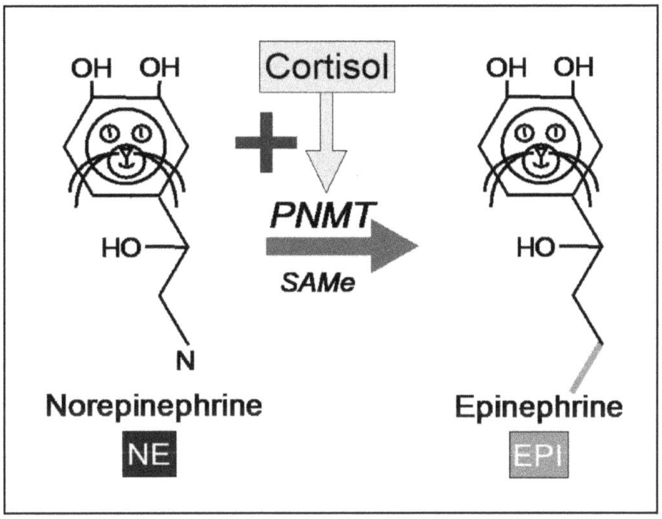

NE is converted to EPI in adrenomedullary cells by the enzyme phenylethanolamine-N-methyltransferase (PNMT). S-adenosylmethionine (SAMe) is the methyl group donor. Cortisol is a trophic factor for PNMT.

The direction of blood flow in the adrenal gland is from the outer shell, the cortex, through the inner portion, the medulla. As a result, adrenomedullary cells normally are bathed in very high concentrations of adrenocortical steroids. Cortisol, the main glucocorticoid in the human adrenal cortex, is trophic for PNMT. This trophism is one piece of evidence for functional links between the cortical and medullary layers of the adrenal "bon-bon."

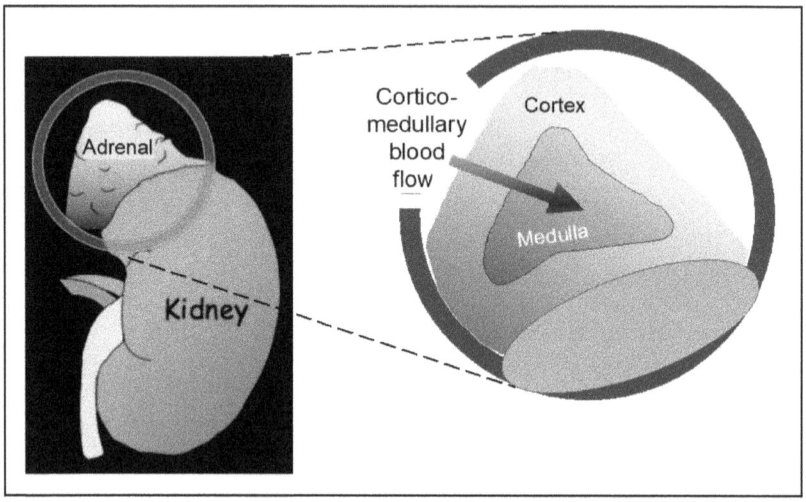

The sympathetic adrenergic system (SAS) seems to be more susceptible than the sympathetic noradrenergic system (SNS) to hormonal influences. In addition to the local effects of the hormone cortisol due to the adrenal "bon-bon" arrangement, the adrenal medulla contains abundant receptors for angiotensin II (AII). AII, one of the key component biochemicals of the renin-angiotensin-aldosterone system (RAS), evokes secretion of catecholamines from adrenomedullary cells.

Exocytosis and the omega sign

A key chemical messaging step in the ANS is release of the neurotransmitters that are stored in the vesicles. The release occurs by a process called exocytosis.

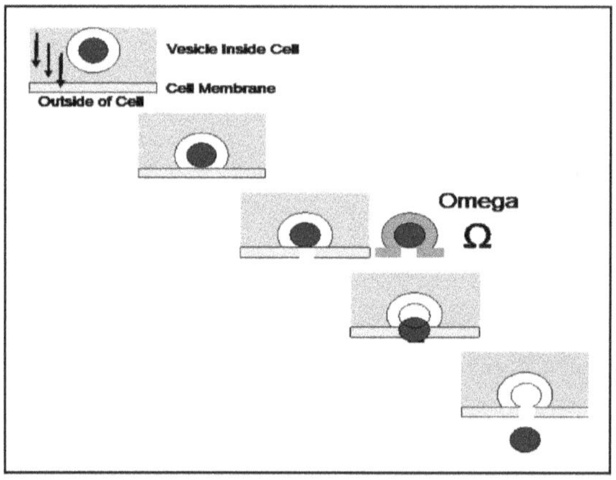

Exocytosis. Poration of the vesicles produces an "omega sign" in electron micrographs.

According to the exocytosis theory, chemical neurotransmission results from physical movement of the bubble-like vesicles containing the neurotransmitter toward the cell membrane, fusion of the vesicle membrane with the cell membrane, pore formation at the site of fusion of the two membranes, and entry of the contents of the vesicles into the fluid outside the cell. Among those contents is the neurotransmitter, which diffuses a short way to reach receptors on the membrane of the target cells.

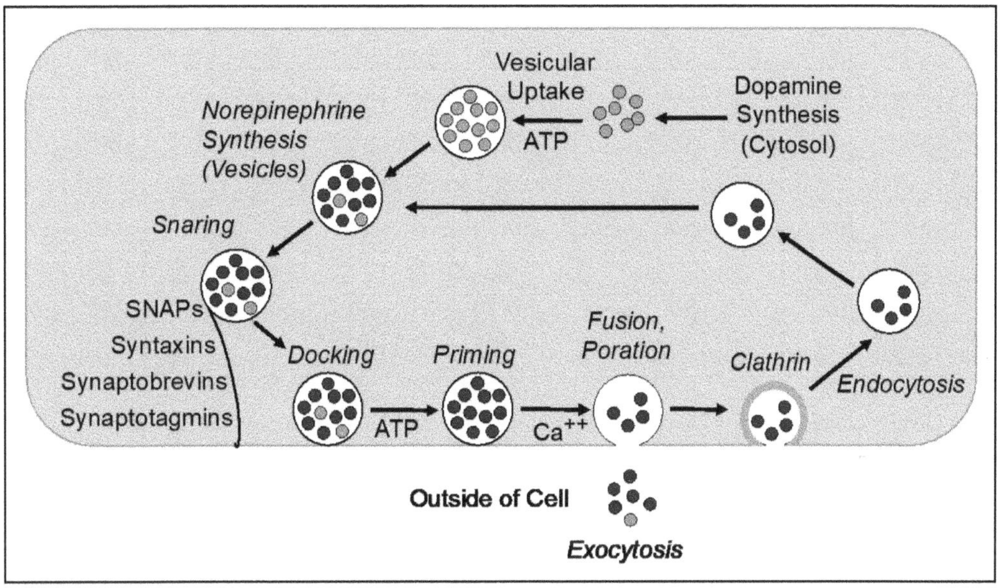

Vesicle docking, exocytosis, and recycling by endocytosis.

Co-transmission

Autonomic neurons and cells can store and release more than one chemical messenger. This means they can have more than one neurochemical "signature," or phenotype, suggesting the notion of biochemical "coding" in the autonomic nervous system. It was not until the 1970s that the concept of co-transmission was proposed formally and became generally accepted. Adenosine triphosphate (ATP) has been reported to be co-released with acetylcholine, the catecholamines, and non-adrenergic, non-cholinergic neurons of the enteric nervous system.

Catecholamine reuptake

After release of catecholamines from nerves, the neurotransmitters undergo inactivation mainly by a conservative recycling process, in which the nerves take back up the released catecholamine. This process has been called Uptake-1. Julius Axelrod introduced the idea that termination of the actions of a neuro-transmitter can occur by neuronal reuptake, as opposed to enzymatic degradation of the NE transmitter in the extracellular fluid (which is the fate of released acetylcholine). For this discovery Axelrod shared (with U.S. von Euler) the Nobel Prize for Physiology or Medicine in 1970.

The neuronal reuptake process is relatively specific for the particular neuro-transmitter. One might even define the type of nerve cell by the neurotrans-mitter it takes up. Uptake-1 involves at least two different transporters, which physically transport the neurotransmitter molecules into the cells. The transporter for NE is the cell membrane norepinephrine transporter, or NET. The transporter for DA is called the dopamine transporter, or DAT. One of the peculiarities of the functioning of these transporters is that DA is more avidly taken up via the NET than NE is.

The NE recycling process is completed by translocation of the NE from the cytoplasm into storage vesicles by the VMAT. Because of the NET, the concentration of NE in the cytoplasm normally exceeds by many-fold that in the extracellular fluid outside sympathetic neurons; and because of the VMAT, the concentration of norepinephrine in the vesicles normally exceeds by many-fold that in the cytoplasm. Since the NET and VMAT act in series, the concentration of NE in the storage vesicles normally is several thousand times the concentration in the extracellular fluid. Now that's recycling!

Catecholamine metabolism

Although catecholamines are recycled quite efficiently in sympathetic nerves, a small percent of the catecholamine in the cytoplasm undergoes metabolic breakdown via a process that is catalyzed by the enzyme monoamine oxidase (MAO). MAO plays a key role in the metabolism of the catecholamines DA and NE.

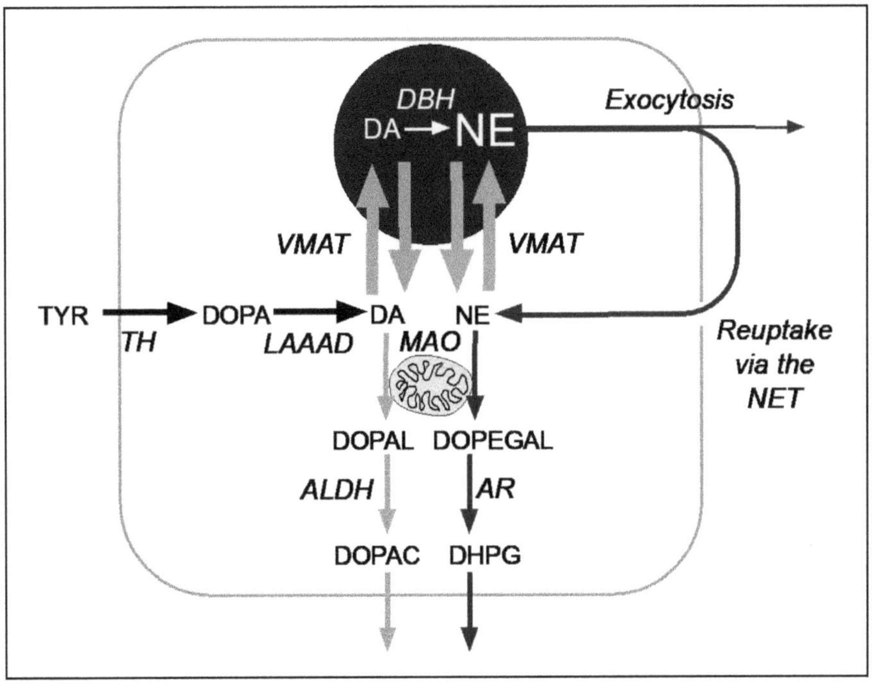

Monoamine oxidase (MAO) in the outer mitochondrial membrane metabolizes cytoplasmic DA and NE.

MAO is found in the outer membrane of the mitochondria, the cell's energy plants.

There are two forms of MAO, MAO-A and MAO-B. The main form in sympathetic nerves is MAO-A. MAO catalyzes the conversion of DA to an aldehyde called DOPAL (an abbreviation for 3,4-dihydroxyphenylacetaldehyde).

Analogously, MAO catalyzes the conversion of NE to an aldehyde called DOPEGAL (an abbreviation for 3,4- dihydroxyphenylglycolaldehyde). As for all aldehydes formed in cells of the body, DOPAL and DOPEGAL are toxic. Their toxicity is the basis for the "catecholaldehyde hypothesis" for the loss of catecholamine-producing neurons that characterizes neurodegenerative diseases such as Parkinson's disease.

Both DOPAL and DOPEGAL are toxic but normally are detoxified by another metabolic step. The enzyme aldehyde dehydrogenase (ALDH) converts DOPAL to the acidic catechol, DOPAC (an abbreviation for 3,4-dihydroxyphenylacetic acid).

The oxidized form of nicotinamide adenine dinucleotide (NAD+) is a required co-factor for ALDH. NAD+ is produced in mitochondria as result of the Complex 1 in the mitochondrial electron "bucket brigade" that results in ATP generation. Drugs such as rotenone, which inhibits Complex 1, indirectly inhibit ALDH activity; a consequence is DOPAL accumulation. Just as DOPAC is the main intra-neuronal metabolite of DA, DHPG is the main intra-neuronal metabolite of NE. DHPG is a glycol (somewhat resembling the body sugar, glucose) that easily passes through cell membranes and enters the circulation.

The ends of the lines

Non-neuronal cells contain the enzyme catechol-O- methyltransferase, or COMT. COMT transfers a methyl group to DOPAC, with S-adenosyl-methionine (SAMe) serving as the methyl group donor, to form homovanillic acid (HVA). HVA is the main end-product of dopamine metabolism.

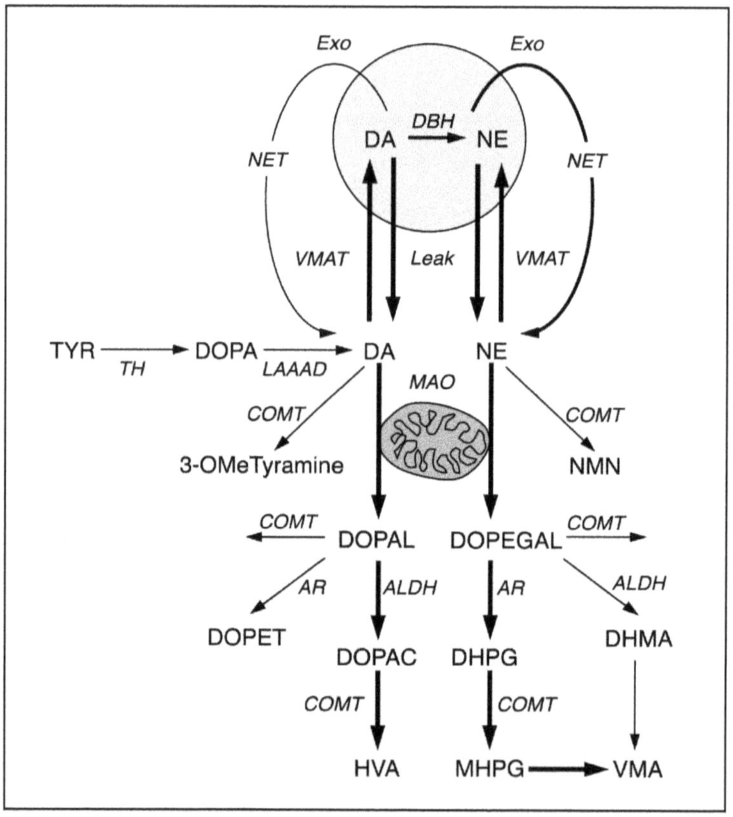

Summary of catecholamine metabolism.

There are two main end-products of NE metabolism—MHPG and VMA. MHPG is an abbreviation for 3-methoxy-4-hydroxyphenylglycol, and VMA is an abbreviation for vanillylmandelic acid. Circulating DHPG is converted extensively to MHPG by COMT. In the liver much of MHPG is converted to VMA.

Norepinephrine turnover

The rate of synthesis of NE in a tissue is normally balanced by the rate of loss of NE and all its metabolites from the tissue (turnover). One might think that the main determinant of tissue NE turnover is exocytotic release with escape of reuptake via the NET. In fact, under resting conditions most of NE turnover is from net leakage from vesicles into the cytoplasm. There are two general reasons for this. First, the NET is so efficient in taking released NE back up into the nerve, relatively little of released NE escapes neuronal reuptake. Second, there is a tremendously high rate of vesicular uptake of NE via the VMAT. There is a correspondingly high rate of passive leakage into the cytoplasm. The enzymatic sequence of MAO and AR acting on cytoplasmic NE then results in DHPG formation.

Dopamine surprises

Most of the synthesis and metabolism of DA in humans takes place not in the brain or in the autonomic nervous system—in fact not in nerves at all—but in non-neuronal cells of the gut. The functions and regulation of this non-neuronal DA system are poorly understood.

Another surprising fact about DA metabolism is that there is a very large amount of DOPAC in the urine—far more than can be accounted for by filtration of DOPAC in the plasma reaching the kidneys. Most of the DA, and probably most of the DOPAC, in the urine comes from uptake and decarboxylation of circulating DOPA by non-neuronal cells in the kidneys, in the renal DOPA-dopamine autocrine/paracrine system.

Virtually all of the DA in the plasma exists not in free form but as a conjugated form—DA sulfate. The conjugation takes place in the gut via an enzyme called monoamine-preferring phenolsulfotransferase (mPST). Catecholamines in a queous solution are extremely susceptible to oxidation. Over the course of hours, a clear solution of DA takes on a tan color, and by the next day there is a black powdery precipitate. This is why a tan color indicates that an EpiPen has expired and should be replaced.

In summarizing catecholamine synthesis and metabolism there are a few general principles to have in mind.

1. DA and NE have a single source, DOPA.
2. DA is made in the cytoplasm, whereas NE is made in the vesicles.
3. Released NE is recycled by uptake into the cytoplasm via the NET followed by uptake into the vesicles via the VMAT.
4. In healthy people, the main determinant of catecholamine turnover under resting conditions is not release by exocytosis followed by extra-neuronal metabolism but rather vesicular leakage followed by MAO.
5. MAO plays a central role in catecholamine metabolism. Virtually all of neuronal catecholamine metabolism occurs via MAO.
6. End-products of catecholamine metabolism are formed in the gut and liver.

Catecholamine receptors

The chemical messengers of the autonomic nervous system exert their effects on body functions by way of receptors and particular "second messengers" in the target organs. Receptors are highly specialized molecules embedded in the membranes of the target cells. The synthesis of chemical messengers and the processes of their metabolism seem relatively simple compared to the bewildering arrays and locations of the receptors. Most drugs used to treat dysautonomias work by way of their effects on receptors.

EPI stimulates all types of adrenoceptors. By way of occupying beta-2 adrenoceptors on vascular smooth muscle cells, EPI indirectly increases release of NE from sympathetic noradrenergic nerves.

NE exerts its cardiovascular effects mainly by stimulating alpha-adrenoceptors.
It also is an agonist at beta-1 adrenoceptors, but, unlike EPI, NE is a relatively poor agonist at beta-2 adrenoceptors.

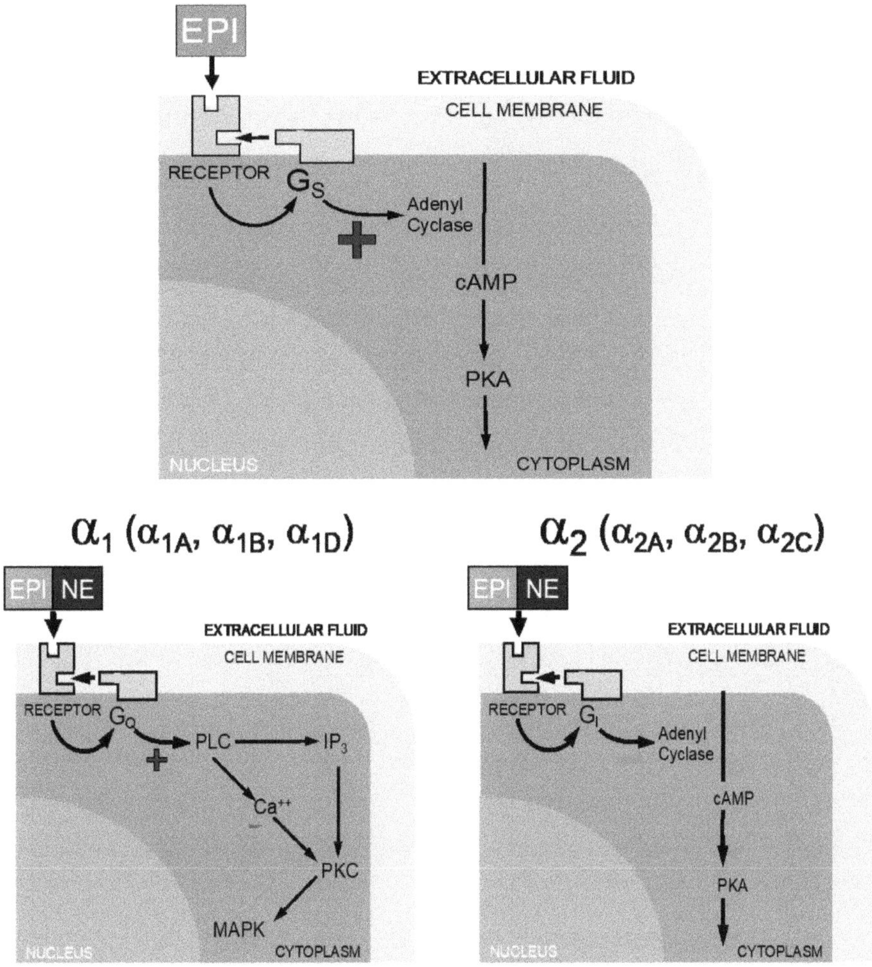

Second messenger systems in target cells mediate effects of receptor occupation by EPI and NE.

In the liver, EPI liberates the vital metabolic fuel, glucose. This is a major way that EPI increases blood glucose levels. The release of glucose by EPI takes place partly by stimulating the breakdown of glycogen to form glucose. The breakdown of glycogen, in turn, involves a rather involved cascade of biochemical events. For this cascade to begin requires the formation of a messenger substance, cyclic adenosine monophosphate (cAMP), inside the liver cells. cAMP was the first identified intracellular messenger, or "second messenger." (The first would be the hormone itself, such as EPI).

For more information about Second Messengers see the full online text.

Acetylcholine

Acetylcholine is the main chemical messenger of two components of the ANS, the parasympathetic nervous system (PNS) and the sympathetic cholinergic system (SCS).

Acetylcholine (ACh) is produced from the action of the enzyme, choline acetyltransferase (ChAT), on choline and acetyl coenzyme A in the neuronal cytoplasm. ChAT catalyzes the transfer of the acetate ion from acetyl coenzyme A to choline.

In the body probably the main role of acetyl coenzyme A is in the Krebs cycle, providing the acetyl group that is oxidized for energy production. Oxidation of the acetyl group yields carbon dioxide, water, and energy that is captured in he form of 11 adenosine triphosphate (ATP) molecules and one guanosine triphosphate (GTP) molecule per acetyl group.

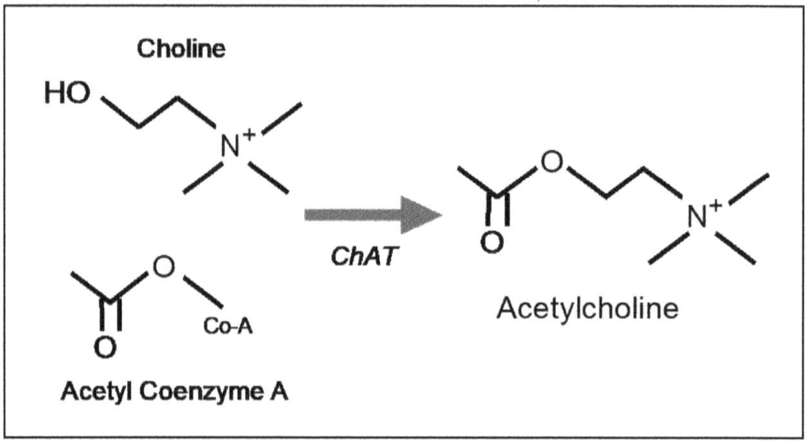

Acetylcholine is formed from the action of choline acetyltransferase (ChAT) on choline and acetyl coenzyme A.

As for other neurotransmitters, ACh formed in the neuronal cytoplasm is actively taken up into vesicles by a transporter, in this case the vesicular acetylcholine transporter, or VAChT. Because ACh is required for neuromuscular transmission, blockade of the VAChT causes skeletal muscle paralysis.

After release of ACh by exocytosis into the extracellular fluid, the transmitter can bind to specific receptors on target cells, but it is also rapidly broken down by the enzyme acetylcholinesterase (AChE), which regenerates the acetate and choline. Because of the rapid breakdown of acetylcholine by AChE, it is impossible to monitor activity of the cholinergic neurons by measuring levels of acetylcholine in body fluids such as plasma or urine.

Cholinergic receptors

The neurotransmitter in all the autonomic ganglia is ACh. Acetylcholine binds to nicotinic receptors on the cell bodies of the post-ganglionic nerves.

There are two classes of receptors for acetylcholine—nicotinic and muscarinic. These names are derived from the drugs nicotine, which is made in tobacco plants, and muscarine, which is made in certain types of mushrooms.

The chemical structures of nicotine and muscarine differ, but they both are small organic molecules that contain prominent nitrogen atoms.

Nicotinic receptors

Nicotine is the classic stimulator of the neuronal nicotinic receptor—the first type of neurotransmitter receptor to be identified.

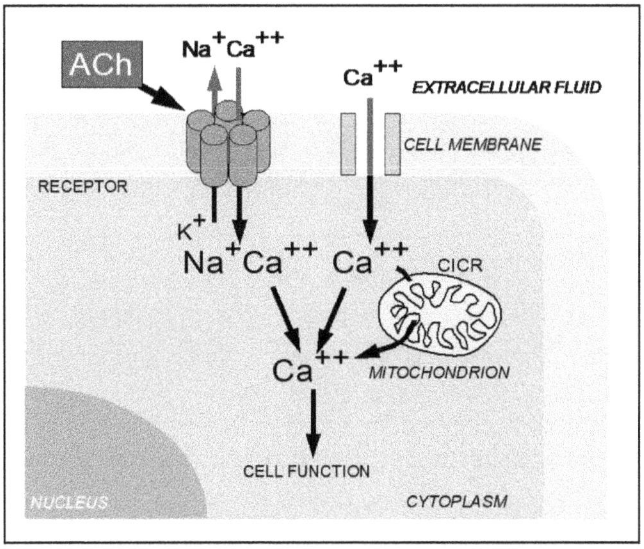

Nicotinic cholinergic receptors are "ionotropic."

Nicotinic receptors are called "ionotropic," because when they are occupied by acetylcholine they allow ions to enter the cell from the extracellular fluid. By letting in sodium ions the cells lose some of their charge (i.e., they depolarize), and the depolarization then enables calcium ions to enter.

Calcium ion builds up in the cell through the channel itself or via induced calcium release from intracellular stores. It is the buildup of ionized calcium in the cytoplasm that activates the cell.

There are numerous types and sub-types of nicotinic receptors. All have 5 component parts—i.e., they are pentamers. For instance, a common arrangement in the sympathetic ganglia is a pentamer that has 2 alpha-3 subunits 3 beta-4 subunits.

The constituents of the nicotinic receptor mediating skeletal muscle neuro-transmission differ from those of the nicotinic receptor mediating ganglionic neurotransmission. This is why ganglion blockade with a neuronal nicotinic receptor blocker does not cause paralysis.

It's a girl!

Stimulation of nicotinic receptors on adrenomedullary cells rapidly evokes EPI release. Here is an anecdote to help remember this fact.

When my brother and sister-in-law had their youngest daughter, they gave me an "It's a Girl!" cigar. I've never been a tobacco smoker, but given the occasion I thought I should smoke it. My wife wouldn't let me smoke in the house, so I decided to take a stroll in the neighborhood around our long block. I lit up and started a leisurely walk, and I was puffing away proudly with my chin high and hands clasped behind my back when about half way around the block I suddenly came to the realization that I was about to die.

My heart was racing, I broke out in a sweat, I gasped for breath, I began to tremble, and I experienced what in medical circles is called the "feeling of impending doom." I made it home and flung myself on the couch in our family room. From my pallor, sweating, hyperventilation, and tremulous speech, everyone was immediately concerned and wanted to know what was wrong. I gasped, "It's that damned It's a Girl! cigar."

All these symptoms and signs were due to release of adrenaline from my adrenal glands after occupation of nicotinic receptors on my adrenomedullary cells.

In non-smokers, the nicotine in tobacco smoke releases adrenaline, producing fast pulse rate, sweating, pallor, hyperventilation, and a "feeling of impending doom."

Muscarinic receptors

Muscarinic receptors for ACh are expressed in virtually all the organs of the body, including the heart, gut, sweat glands, urinary bladder, and lungs. Probably the most noticeable effect of muscarinic receptor stimulation is gastrointestinal upset, nausea, and vomiting.

Of the five types of muscarinic receptors, the M2 type is the main form in the heart. Stimulation of the M2 receptors in the heart decreases the rate and force of heart contraction, via two processes.

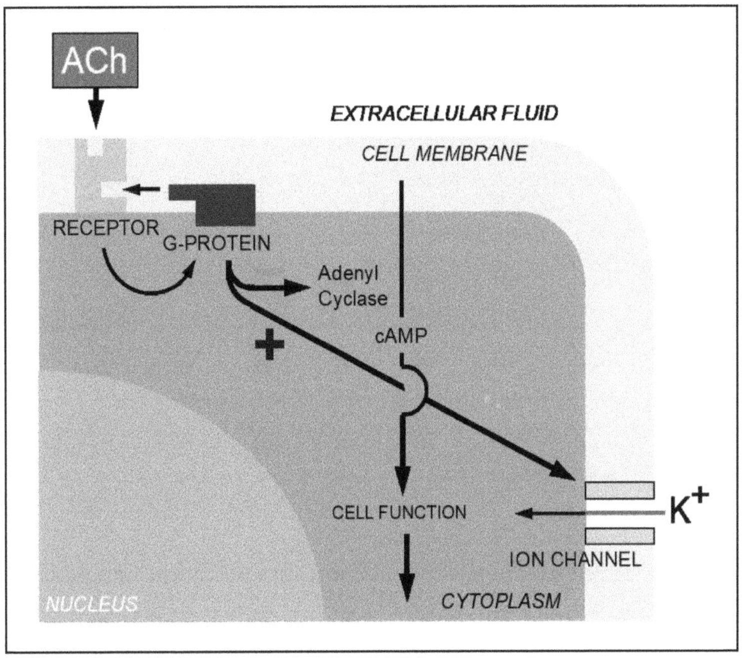

Muscarinic cholinergic receptors are "metabotropic."

First, occupation of M2 receptors on the heart muscle cells inhibits the cells' activities via decreasing generation of the second messenger cyclic AMP and augmenting the entry of potassium ion into the cells. Second, stimulation of M2 receptors on cardiac sympathetic nerves inhibits NE release for a given amount of post-ganglionic sympathetic nerve traffic.

Another cholinergic signaling system mediates relaxation of blood vessels independently of muscarinic receptors. This system involves production of the gas, nitric oxide (NO).

NO is generated in different types of cells. In this case we are dealing with NO production within the endothelial cells that line the innermost walls of blood vessels. NO diffuses from the endothelial cells to nearby smooth muscle cells, causing the smooth muscle cells to relax.

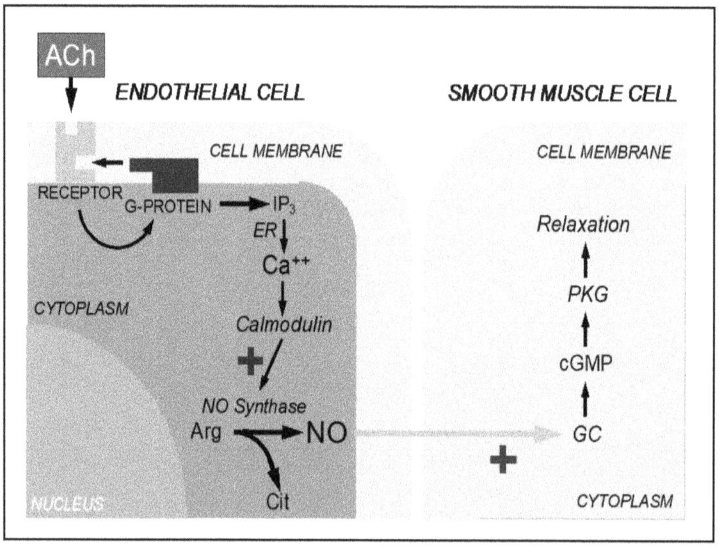

Occupation of cholinergic receptors can evoke release of nitric oxide (NO), resulting in vascular relaxation.

The acetylcholine/NO mechanism plays an important role in the relaxation of local blood vessels in the corpora cavernosa that enables blood to engorge the penis during erection. When this pair of sponge-like structures fill with blood, their expansion interferes with venous return of blood in the shaft, and the penis stiffens.

Neurotrophic factors

Release of NE in response to traffic in sympathetic nerves depends on the existence of functional sympathetic nerve terminals. The development and continued existence of sympathetic nerves in an organ depend in turn on a continuous supply of a nerve growth factor.

Since the discovery of NGF a variety of other neurotrophic factors have been described, such as glial cell line-derived neurotrophic factor (GDNF) and brain-derived neurotrophic factor (BDNF).

According to the "neurotrophic factor hypothesis," neuronal survival requires target-derived factors. The neurotrophic factors themselves, membrane receptors for the factors, or second messengers produced by neurotrophic receptor occupation are transmitted retrogradely in the axons to the neuronal cell bodies, promoting neuronal growth, axonal sprouting, and survival. Experimental data about NGF fit with the neurotrophic factor hypothesis. For instance, after injection of a radiolabeled NGF into axon terminals radioactivity is detected in neuronal cell bodies.

HOMEOSTASIS, STRESS, AND THE ANS

The 19th century French physiologist Claude Bernard introduced the idea of the "inner world" inside the body—what he called the milieu intérieur. He theorized that a constant fluid environment bathes all the body's cells. Near the end of his life, in about 1876, he postulated something even more profound. The body maintains the constant internal environment by myriad, continual, compensatory reactions. These compensatory reactions tend to restore a state of equilibrium in response to any outside changes and in so doing enable independence of the organism from the vicissitudes of the external environment. Bernard therefore not only introduced the notion of an apparently constant inner world but also a purpose for body processes.

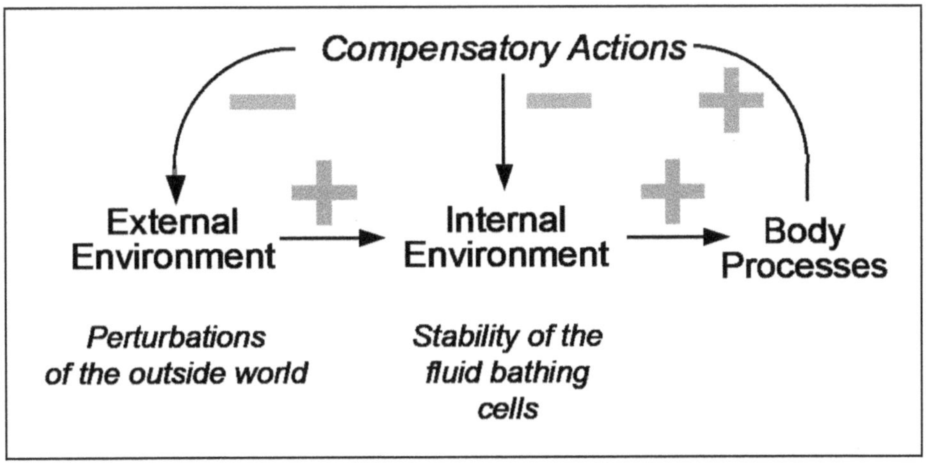

According to Claude Bernard, a variety of body processes maintain the stability of the fluid bathing cells, the internal environment, or what he called the milieu intérieur.

The (+) signs in the concept diagram indicate stimulatory effects, and the (-) signs indicate inhibitory effects. Loops with single (-) signs maintain stability. A perturbation of the outside world has an effect on the internal environment, but the internal environmental changes evoke effects on body processes that act compensatorily on the external or internal environments. It can be shown mathematically that in any system containing a negative feedback loop, the level of the monitored variable reaches a stable, plateau level.

Bernard wrote, "The constancy of the internal environment is the condition for free and independent life...All the vital mechanisms, however varied they might be, always have one purpose, that of maintaining the integrity of the conditions of life within the internal environment. "This view may seem obvious now, but it was revolutionary in the history of medical ideas.

Bernard's visionary concept of the stability of the internal environment attracted little attention until Walter B. Cannon proposed his theory of homeostasis.

Cannon's "homeostasis"

Cannon coined the word, "homeostasis." He used this term to describe the overall stability of the various constituents of body fluids and of core temperature that make up the body's inner world. The full description of this new concept was based on the results of Cannon's own studies and those reported in the two decades preceding his 1929 review, "Organization for Physiological Homeostasis."

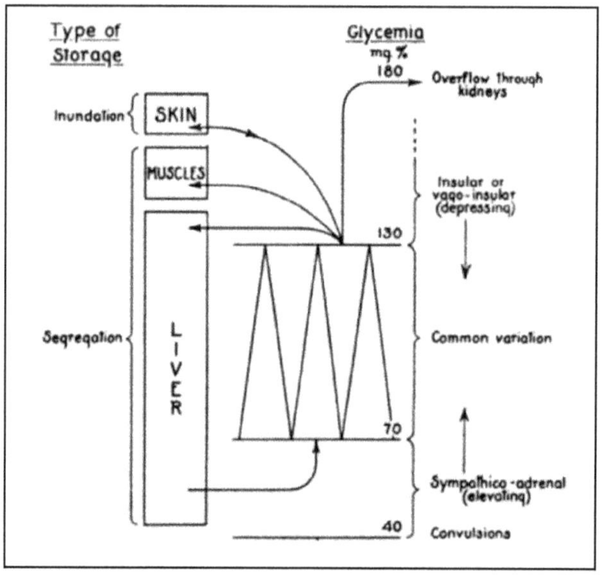

Cannon's classic presentation of his theory in 1929 in Physiological Reviews contains one diagram.

According to Cannon, the blood glucose level ("glycemia") is kept within bounds, because when the glucose level goes down the "sympathico-adrenal" system (in this book called the sympathetic adrenergic system, or SAS) is activated. This activation increases the glucose level via the stimulatory effects of high circulating adrenaline levels on the liver, releasing glucose into the bloodstream. When the glucose level goes down the vago-insular system (in this book the parasympathetic nervous system, or PNS) is activated, and this decreases the glucose level via the stimulatory effects of acetylcholine on insulin secretion by the pancreas, augmenting cellular uptake of circulating glucose.

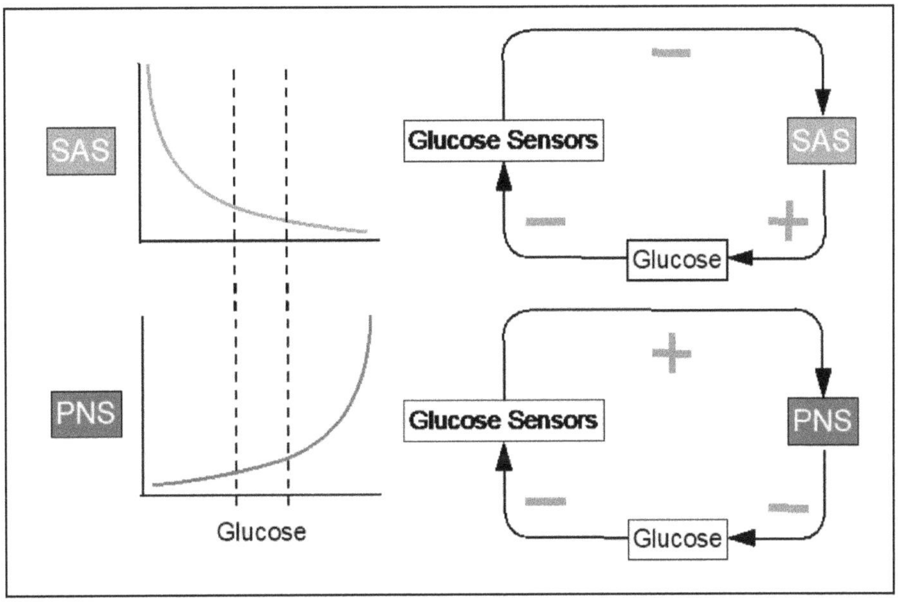

Homeostasis of blood glucose by opposing negative feedback loops.

Similar sorts of diagrams can be drawn for homeostasis of core temperature via the SNS and SAS (activation of which tends to increase temperature by decreasing blood flow to the skin, thereby decreasing evaporative heat loss) and SCS (activation of which tends to decrease temperature by augmenting sweating and thereby increasing evaporative heat loss).

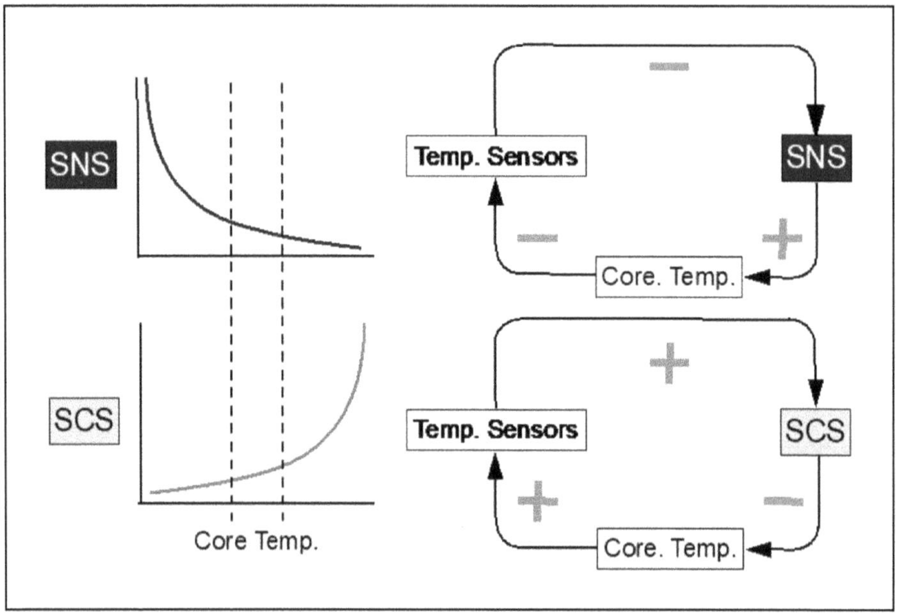

Homeostasis of blood glucose by opposing negative feedback loops.

From teleology to homeostats

Teleology is a doctrine that explains phenomena in terms of their purpose, goal, or end. The word comes for the Greek, telos, meaning "end," and logos, meaning "reason."

Teleology has had a checkered past in science. Physics and chemistry discarded teleology centuries ago, but it remains an unsettled aspect of biology. Integrative physiologists often think teleologically. When they ponder the function of a body process, they have in mind the purpose of that process. In contrast, when systems biologists think about the function of a body process, they have in mind the mechanism.

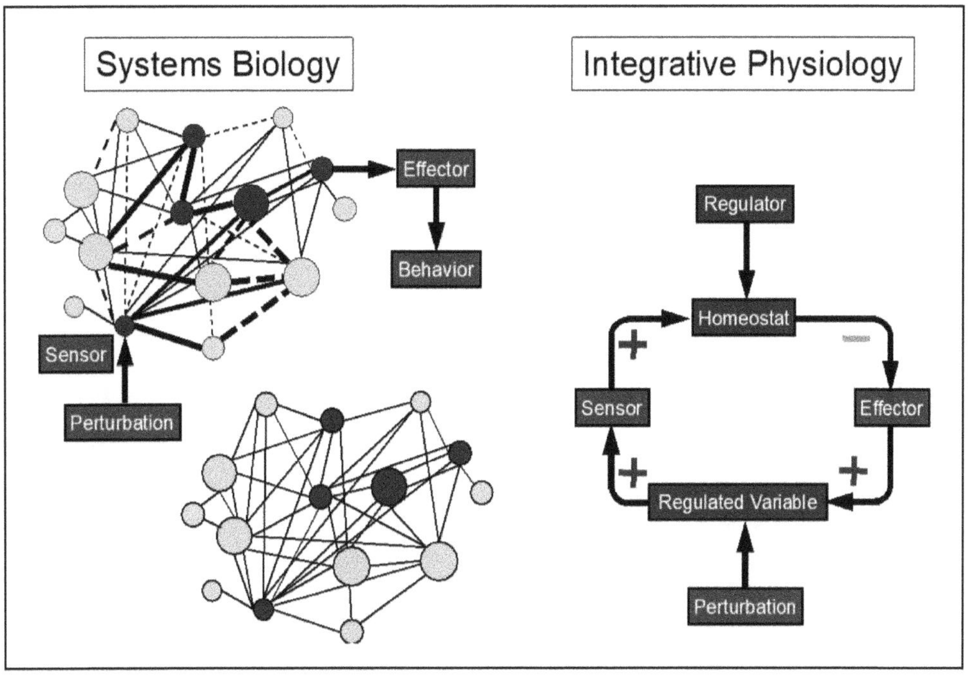

Systems biological and integrative physiological models. In system biology homeostasis is an outcome. In integrative physiology homeostasis is a goal.

In the systems biology model depicted on the left, homeostasis is an emergent phenomenon resulting from a pattern of activation (thick solid lines) and inhibition (thick dashed lines) among positive (solid lines) and negative relationships (dashed lines) embedded in a network. Homeostasis is not a goal; it is simply a fact emerging from the operations of complex networks. In integrative physiology, homeostasis is a key goal driving body processes.

In the integrative physiology model, there is a negative feedback loop that keeps levels of the regulated variable within bounds. There is a "regulator" that provides an algorithm for responding to a homeostatic comparator, a "homeostat." Information about a "regulated variable" (e.g., core temperature) reaches the homeostat, which compares the sensed information with the algorithm for responding, and the discrepancy (error signal) determines the state of activity of an effector (e.g., the sympathetic noradrenergic system).

Homeostats

Homeostats are metaphorical comparators that work like thermostats. For a given perturbation, the more rapid, sensitive, and powerful the control by negative feedback, the smaller the fluctuations in levels of the monitored variable. When a system regulated by negative feedback is exposed to a fluctuating outside influence, the swings in the levels of the monitored variable are smaller than in the absence of negative feedback. Combined heating and cooling systems, each controlled by a single thermostat that can turn on either the furnace or the air conditioner, constitute a thermostatic system.

One can think of a multitude of internal homeostatic systems, each with its own "homeostat"—a "barostat" for regulating blood pressure, a "thermostat" for regulating core temperature, a "glucostat" for regulating blood glucose levels, an "osmostat" for regulating serum osmolality, and so forth. This of course introduces a problem: homeostats, regulators, and regulated variables are all ideas. We are dealing here with metaphors. They cannot be observed directly. Their existence cannot be disproven, which makes them weak scientifically.

Nevertheless, thinking in terms of homeostatic systems can yield valuable insights and organizing concepts, such as stress and allostasis, which are covered later in this section.

This section develops the idea that homeostasis does not result from negative feedback alone. Instead, three types of process maintain homeostasis. The first and most well-known is error control by negative feedback regulation. The second is feed-forward regulation, which is the most challenging from a theoretical point of view. The third is buffering.

The concept diagram on the next page shows the relationships of reflexive error control via negative feedback, buffering, and anticipatory regulation. The anticipatory control mechanisms can be instinctive (solid lines) or conditioned (dashed lines). A disturbance can arouse anticipatory instinctive responses by pathways involving awareness (conscious or unconscious); and an associated conditioned stimulus can arouse anticipatory responses by pathways involving awareness and conditioned learning. A disturbance is sensed by interoceptors (e.g., gastrointestinal hemorrhage) or exteroceptors (e.g., touching a hot iron), while a conditioned stimulus is sensed by exteroceptors.

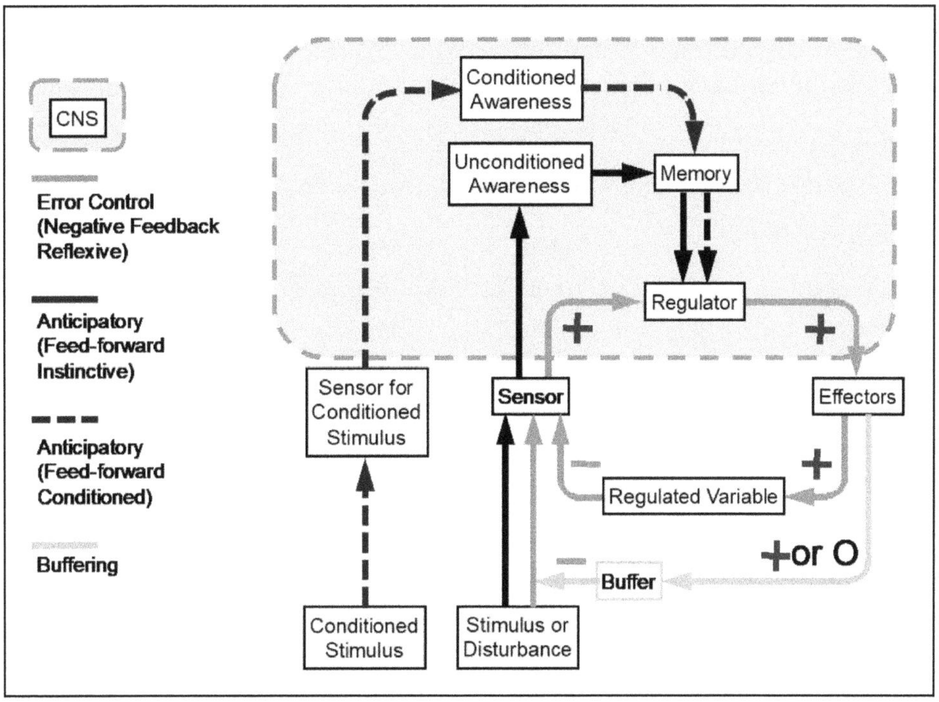

Three ways homeostasis is maintained—negative feedback, feed-forward anticipatory behaviors, and buffering.

Examples of negative feedback regulation abound in autonomic medicine. For instance, insulin-induced hypoglycemia, via a complex network of peripheral and central mechanisms, evokes marked sympathetic adrenergic system (SAS) activation and adreno-medullary secretion of epinephrine (EPI), which releases glucose into the bloodstream. Performance of the Valsalva maneuver, which decreases venous return to the heart and consequently decreases cardiac stroke volume, reflexively increases skeletal muscle SNS traffic and total peripheral vascular resistance, attenuating the fall in blood pressure.

Intravenous injection of cold saline evokes increases in both SNS and SAS and outflows, resulting in cutaneous vasoconstriction and calorigenesis that blunt the fall in core temperature. Standing up (orthostasis) decreases venous return to the heart, and this rapidly increases SNS outflow via low-pressure and arterial baroreceptors.

Multiple effectors & shared effectors

Two principles of homeostat operation are multiple effectors and shared effectors.

Having multiple effectors extends the range of control of the monitored variable, enables compensatory activation of alternative effectors if one is disabled, and provides a basis for stressor-specific patterning.

Examples of compensatory activation are increased sympathetic noradrenergic system (SNS) activity in the setting of hypothyroidism, SNS activation by adrenalectomies, or decreased activity of the hypothalamic-pituitary-adrenocortical axis.

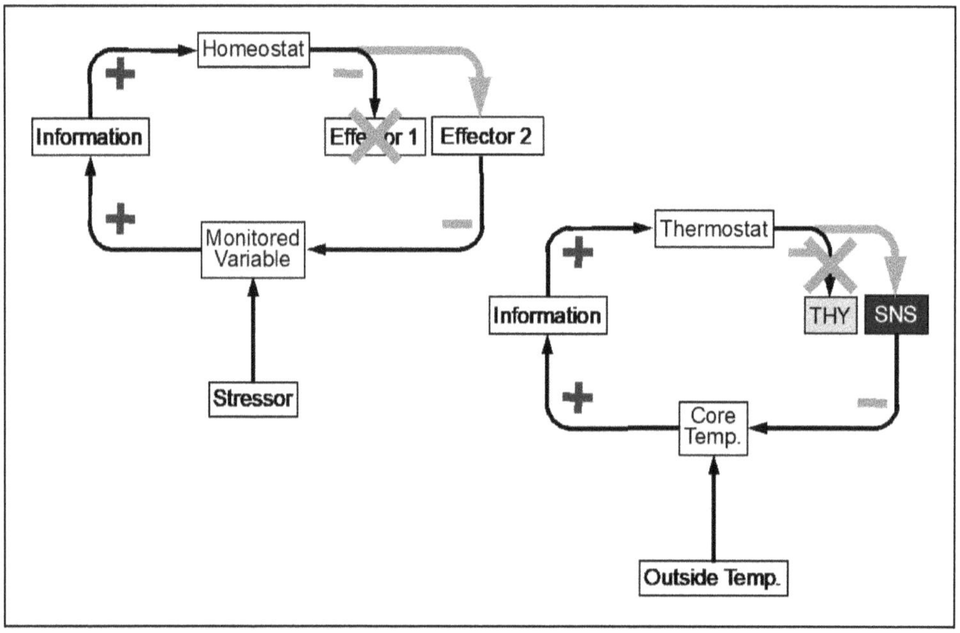

Hypothyroidism increases activity of the sympathetic noradrenergic system (SNS), an example of compensatory activation.

Sharing of the same effector by multiple homeostats can explain a variety of clinical phenomena, such as hyperglycemia in hemorrhagic shock and hyponatremia in decompensated congestive heart failure. The SAS is an effector for both the volustat regulating cardiac filling, with afferents from low-pressure baroreceptors, and the glucostat regulating blood glucose, with afferent input to the brain by circulating glucose. The appropriate treatment of hyperglycemia in hemorrhagic shock would not be insulin administration but stopping the bleeding and transfusion of blood. Arginine vasopressin (AVP) is a shared effector for the barostat and osmostat. The appropriate treatment of hyponatremia in decompensated congestive heart failure would not be infusion of hypertonic saline (which would worsen the heart failure) but treatment of the heart failure, such as by afterload reduction.

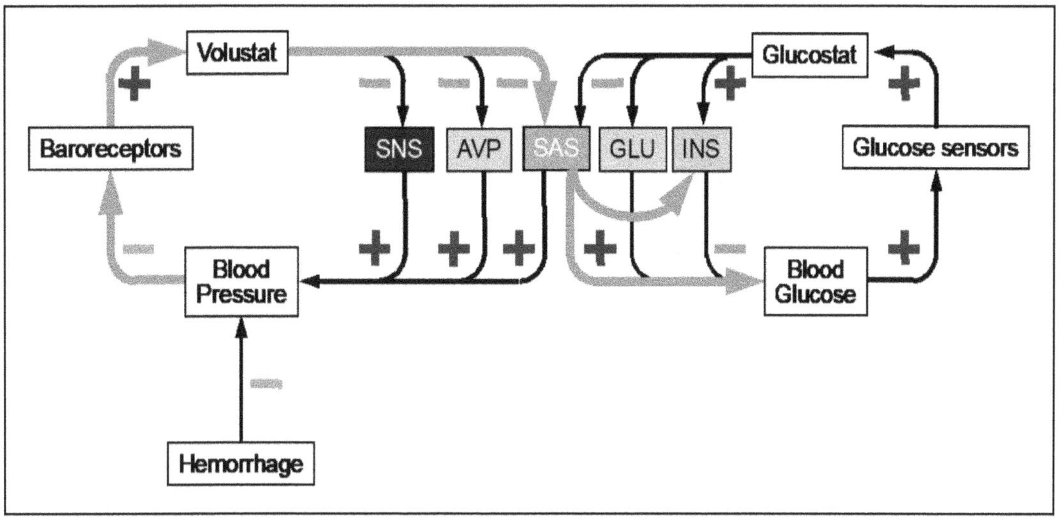

Sharing of the sympathetic adrenergic system (SAS) by the volustat and glucostat explains hyperglycemia in hemorrhagic shock.

Anticipatory (feed-forward) regulation

Regulation by negative feedback is essentially reactive. In contrast, feed-forward regulation is mediated by anticipatory adjustments in physiological systems based on awareness of a previously experienced or instinctively recognized signal, preceding any change in the level of the regulated variable itself.

Feed-forward regulation is more efficient than negative feedback regulation, because it diminishes or eliminates the need for homeostatic adjustments.

An example is vagal mediation of the "cephalic phase" of insulin release prior to eating, in anticipation of an increase in blood glucose.

Another is the pattern of sympathetically mediated hemodynamic changes from "central command" in anticipation of exercise.

Cannon was referring to feed-forward mechanisms when he noted that internal changes during emotional turmoil prepare the organism for extreme muscular exertion.

Anticipatory control usually is learned and is mediated by or associated with externally observable behaviors (i.e., the somatic nervous system). In contrast, error control is reflexive, mediated by effectors such as components of the autonomic nervous system, and may not be associated with externally observable behaviors.

Under normal circumstances, in response to anticipation of environmental challenges (e.g., going out into the cold outdoors) levels of regulated variables are kept within bounds mainly by anticipatory behaviors (e.g., donning a jacket), the elicitation of which depend on input from exteroceptors (e.g., visual input), perception of the meaning of the input (e.g., awareness that snow is falling), and memory (when snow falls, the temperature is cold). The behavior prevents exposure to the environmental challenge from actually altering levels of the regulated variable, the core temperature.

When anticipatory, learned behaviors to deal with cold exposure are insufficient and an actual change in the level of core temperature occurs, the situation evokes reflexive increases in sympathetic noradrenergic and adrenergic outflows, which by cutaneous vasoconstriction and calorigenesis help maintain core temperature. The reflexive responses may include certain externally observable behaviors, such as shivering, piloerection, and folding the arms. In distress, awareness and memory result not only in behaviors (e.g., flight) but also in changes in reflexive regulation (dashed lines.)

Buffering

Buffering is a means of diminishing the intensity of an external disturbance, thereby reducing the required use of reflexive homeostatic mechanisms. Just as insulation in the walls of a house diminishes the requirement of internal adjustment by a furnace in cold weather, many mammals have fur, which creates a layer of motionless air as an insulator above the skin. Other examples of genetically determined insulation include blubber in whales and closely packed feathers in birds. The barrier to heat loss can be enhanced during more severe cold exposure by reflexive bristling of the hair, mediated by sympathetic nerves; this increases the depth of the layer of motionless air.

In addition to these inherited and acquired forms of buffering, countercurrent heat exchange is a relatively common, efficient mechanism in animals that limits heat loss through the surfaces of the body exposed to an extremely cold environment (polar regions or ice cold water). The preservation of heat is the result of differences in the temperature in closely adjacent arterial and venous blood vessels. Heat from arterial blood warms the cold venous blood returning from the cold surface, diminishing heat loss from the surfaces exposed to the cold. This arrangement occurs in the feet of penguins standing on ice and of wading birds in cold water, the paws of the arctic fox, and the tongue of the whale filtering plankton in cold water. The heat transfer between the countercurrent flows depends on the difference in the temperatures and does not require energy other than that required to maintain the flows.

Roles of the brain in homeostasis

In higher organisms, maintaining homeostasis depends on complex coordination by the brain. Just as the brain receives information from sense organs about our interactions with the outside world, the brain also receives information from internal sensors and acts on that information to regulate the inner world. For most of our lives the brain tracks many monitored variables by way of internal sensory information and acts on that information to maintain levels of monitored variables by modulating numerous effectors that work in parallel.

Catecholamines in the central nervous system

Until about the 1950s, dompamine (DA) had been assumed not to have any specific function in the body beyond serving as a chemical intermediary in the production of EPI and NE.

Catecholamines in the brain are found in two NE and three DA pathways and in specific clusters of brainstem and hypothalamic neurons. Different functions of DA have been proposed in its three chemical pathways.

The nigrostriatal system is the main source of DA in the brain and the main determinant of DA effects on movement. Nerve fibers in this system travel from pigmented cells in the substantia nigra ("black substance") in the midbrain portion of the brainstem to much larger structures toward the middle front of the brain. These structures are collectively called the "basal ganglia."

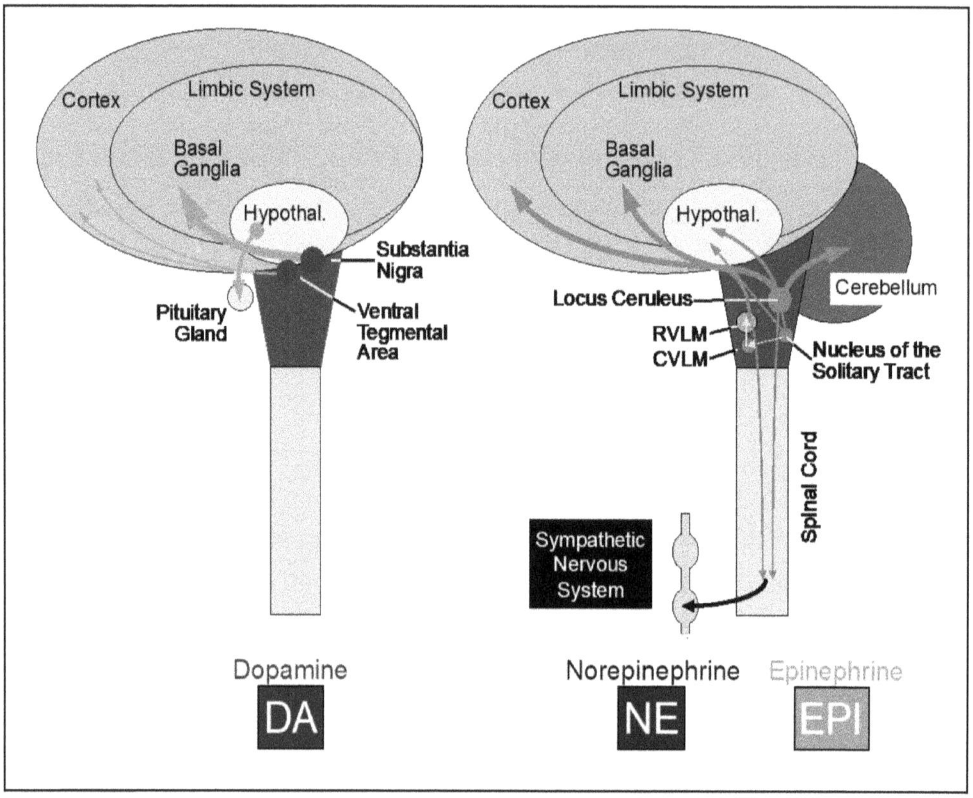

Catecholamine systems in the brain.

The corpus striatum, often simply called the striatum, consists of the caudate and putamen. Loss of DA in the striatum (especially the putamen) produces the movement disorder that defines Parkinson's disease.

The mesolimbic (or mesocortical or mesolimbocortical) system sends DA fibers from the ventral tegmental area (VTA) in the midbrain to the nucleus accumbens and then to other parts of the limbic system, such as the hippocampus and amygdala, and to parts of the cortex, such as the anterior cingulate cortex and pre-frontal cortex. It is thought that this system is dysfunctional in schizophrenia, because many effective drugs for schizophrenia appear to work by blocking the effects of DA in this system. In the mesolimbic system, DA seems to increase locomotion and positive reinforcement, not so much due to pleasurable reward sensations as due to an enabling action that decreases the threshold for initiating responses. Functional alterations of the mesolimbic system are associated with all known forms of addiction.

The tuberoinfundibular (or tuberohypophyseal) system delivers DA from cells in the hypothalamus to the pituitary gland. DA in the pituitary gland inhibits production of prolactin. In postpartum women who don't want to breast-feed, a single injection of bromocriptine, which stimulates DA receptors, prevents lactation.

Complete destruction of all DA systems in the brain produces a syndrome of decreased movement, inattention, decreased food intake, and decreased fluid intake and gives the appearance of generalized behavioral unresponsiveness. This "dopamine deficiency syndrome" applies to all voluntary acts requiring motivation, sustained alertness, and receptiveness to sensory input. Animals deficient in DA fail to initiate coordinated movements and fail to orient to sensory stimuli.

Motivated behaviors are not eliminated, but the arousal threshold appears to be increased before the behaviors are elicited. Most of the research in this area has depended on administration of a neurotoxin to produce chemical destruction of DA cells and terminals; however, the same neurotoxin also destroys noradrenergic cells and terminals.

Increased occupation of DA receptors in the brain, such as produced by DOPA, amphetamines, or drugs that stimulate DA receptors directly, produces hyperactivity, stereotyped involuntary movements, agitation, psychosis, and risk taking. Patients with Parkinson's disease who take DA receptor stimulants can have a surprisingly high frequency of an unusual but related side effect—gambling.

Norepinephrine (NE) also is an established neurotransmitter in the brain, although much less is known about what exactly it does in humans. Based on studies in animals, rather than acting as a direct inhibitor or stimulator of neuronal function, NE seems to modify responsiveness to other inputs. Activation of the locus ceruleus, the brainstem source of most of the NE in the brain, biases attention toward novel, rapidly changing signals from sense organs monitoring both the outside and inner worlds. NE in the locus ceruleus system may therefore play a role in vigilance behavior and in registration of distressing events in long-term memory.

A descending pathway from brainstem NE- producing neurons down the spinal cord seems to contribute to "stress-induced analgesia." If you've ever played in an athletic competition involving repeated bouts of running and noticed painful foot blisters after the game is over, you know what stress-induced analgesia is.

Lower in the brainstem, NE-producing cells participate in neurocirculatory reflexes. Most of the evidence for such a role comes from studies of the baroreflex in laboratory animals. NE-producing cells are abundant in the nucleus of the solitary tract (NTS), which is the site of termination of input from the baroreceptors to the brain. From the NTS, nerve fibers branch widely as they ascend to higher levels of the central nervous system, such as the hypothalamus and amygdala. Conversely, as part of coordinated behavioral, emotional, and autonomic nervous system responses, descending pathway traffic in fibers from higher centers to the NTS can "reset the barostat" and redefine "normal" blood pressure. A loss of NE-producing cells in the NTS can help explain why some neurodegenerative diseases feature extreme swings of blood pressure.

Despite the fact that both DA and NE are known neurotransmitters in the brain, and despite the apparent involvement of dopamine systems and norepinephrine systems in responses to a variety of environmental and internal inputs, interactions between DA systems and NE systems have received relatively little research attention, especially in humans.

The rostral ventrolateral medulla (RVLM) includes neurons called C1 neurons that contain the enzyme PNMT, which catalyzes the conversion of NE to EPI. C1 neurons therefore are thought to be adrenergic. RVLM neurons are a major source of descending projections to the sympathetic pre-ganglionic neurons in the intermediolateral columns of the spinal cord. They also project rostrally to the paraventricular nucleus of the hypothalamus. According to one view, the C1 neurons are the "body's EMTs" because of their involvement with emergency responses to pain, infection, blood loss, hypoxia, and hypoglycemia —analogous to the sympathetic adrenergic system in the periphery.

Neurophysiological studies demonstrated that pre-ganglionic sympathetic neurons discharge rhythmically. The rhythmic discharges depend importantly on lower brainstem networks including coupled oscillators that inherently generate the rhythm—a pacemaker for sympathoneural outflow.

The central autonomic network

Several cortical, subcortical, and brainstem centers in a network participate in regulation of outflows to the autonomic nervous system. This has been called the "central autonomic network."

Cortical centers include the prefrontal cortex, anterior cingulate cortex, and insular cortex. Subcortical centers include the central nucleus of the amygdala and the paraventricular nucleus of the hypothalamus.

Brainstem centers include the peri-aqueductal gray (PAG) region in the midbrain, the parabrachial nucleus (PBN) at the junction of the midbrain and pons, the locus ceruleus (LC) in the dorsal pons, the raphe nuclei, rostral ventrolateral medulla (RVLM), caudal ventrolateral medulla (CVLM), dorsal motor nucleus of the vagus (DMNX), nucleus ambiguus (NA), and the nucleus of the solitary tract (NTS) in the medulla.

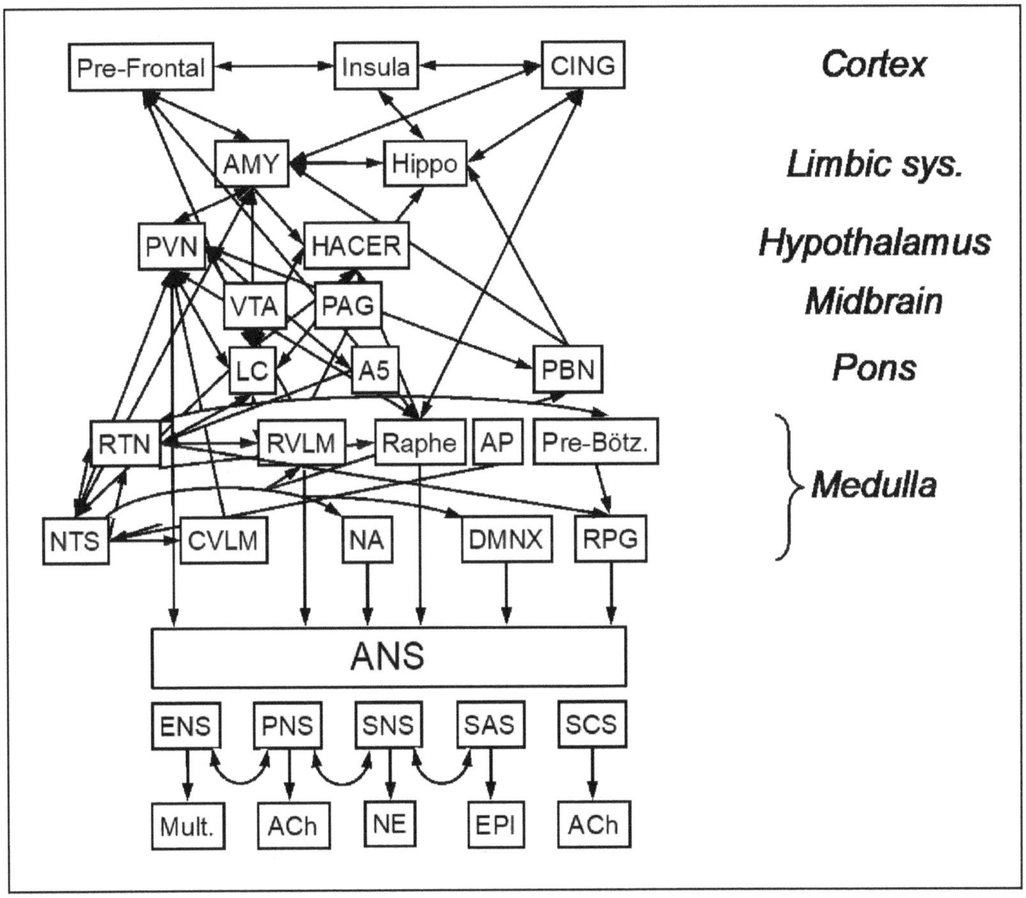

Overview of the central autonomic network.

Although the central autonomic system is defined largely anatomically, different components are also connected by neurochemical pathways, including those that are catecholaminergic.

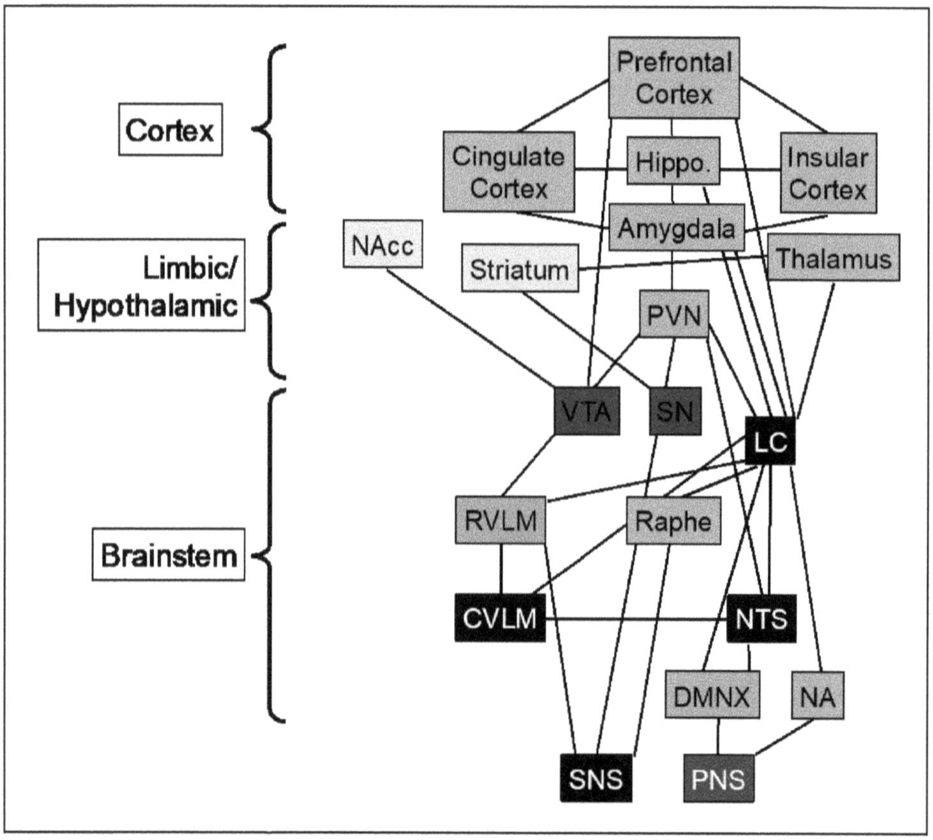

Catecholaminergic pathways in the central autonomic network.

Cortical restraint and the hypothalamus

Cannon studied not only peripheral autonomic systems but also sites in the brain that regulate them. In the 1920s he noted that removal of the cerebral cortices evoked rage behavior, accompanied by high blood glucose levels. Decorticated adrenalectomized animals exhibited the same behavior, but without hyperglycemia. These findings fit with cortical restraint of primitive emotional behaviors and of emotion-associated adrenaline release. Cannon's student, Philip Bard, obtained evidence that physiological concomitants of primitive emotions originate in the hypothalamus.

In the 1920s and 1930s the Swiss physiologist Walter Rudolf Hess focused on the functional organization of the hypothalamus with respect to the regulation of parasympathetic and sympathetic outflows.

Hess showed that stimulation of the same hypothalamic sites that altered functions of internal organs via sympathetic outflows (pupillary dilation, hair bristling, and tachycardia) also evoked particular behaviors that seemed to be directed outwards towards the environment ("ergotropic" effects). In contrast, stimulation of other sites evoked slow heart rate, salivation, pupillary constriction, vomiting, urination, and defecation, consistent with generalized parasympathetic activation. These autonomic effects also were associated with particular behaviors (e.g., postural change associated with defecation).

Hess viewed these changes as protection against a kind of internal overloading ("trophotropic"). The sympathetic- ergotropic and parasympathetic-trophotropic areas operated as if they were in a dynamic state of equilibrium. For this work, Hess received a Nobel Prize in 1949.

Baroreflexes

The term "baroreflex" refers to a rapid reflex where an increase in blood pressure sensed by the brain leads to the relaxation of blood vessels and a decrease in heart rate. The baroreflex keeps blood pressure stable.

Cannon never referred to homeostasis of any cardiovascular variables. Since his time, however, regulation of blood pressure by negative feedback and other studies involving the cardiovascular system have become a major topic of research in autonomic medicine.

Specialized distortion receptors called baroreceptors lie in the carotid sinus, in the crotch of the "Y" where the common carotid arteries, the main arteries delivering lood to the head, fork in the upper neck. When the blood pressure increases, the wall of the carotid sinus on each side of the neck expands, and this stimulates the baroreceptors in the artery walls.

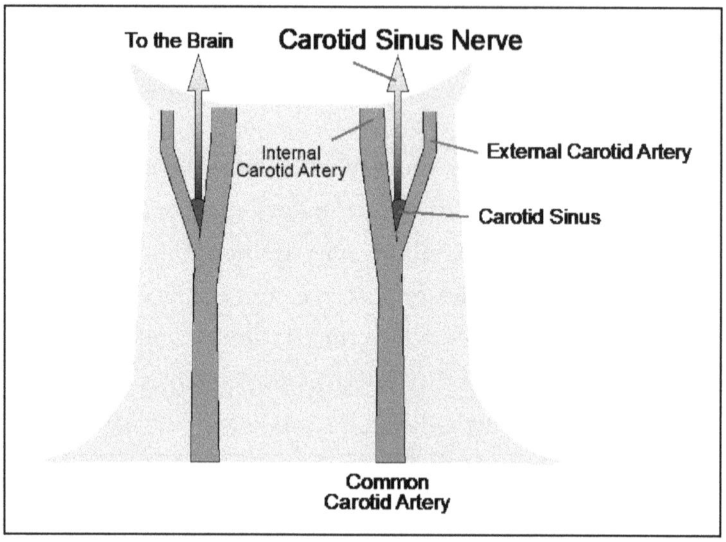

Carotid sinus distortion receptors called baroreceptors send afferent information to the brainstem.

Nerve traffic to the brain then increases in the carotid sinus nerves and reaches a particular cluster of cells in the lower brainstem—the nucleus of the solitary tract, or NTS.

Activation of the NTS cells leads to a rapid, reflexive fall in pulse rate, relaxation of blood vessels, and a less forceful heartbeat. The blood pressure and consequently the blood flow to the brainstem decreases, and the victim loses consciousness.

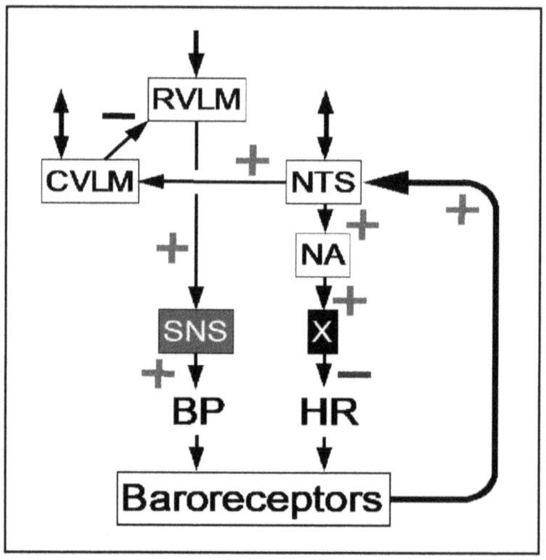

Medullary pathways involved in the arterial baroreflex.

Stimulation of the carotid sinus baroreceptors reflexively decreases sympathetic noradrenergic system (SNS) outflows. This tends to relax the blood vessels and decrease the force and rate of the heartbeat. At about the same time, parasympathetic nervous system (PNS) outflow to the heart via the vagus nerve increases. This also tends to decrease the rate and force of heart contraction. The net effect is to bring the blood pressure down.

The arterial baroreflex involves several other effectors in addition to the SNS and PNS. A sustained decrease in blood pressure releases the arginine vasopressin (AVP) and renin- angiotensin-aldosterone (RAS) systems from baroreceptor restraint.

There are also distortion sensors in low pressure regions such as the atria and pulmonary veins. When a person stands up there is a decrease in venous return to the heart. The "low-pressure baroreceptors" also send afferent nerve fibers to the NTS in the medulla, arousing reflexive changes in outflows in multiple effectors.

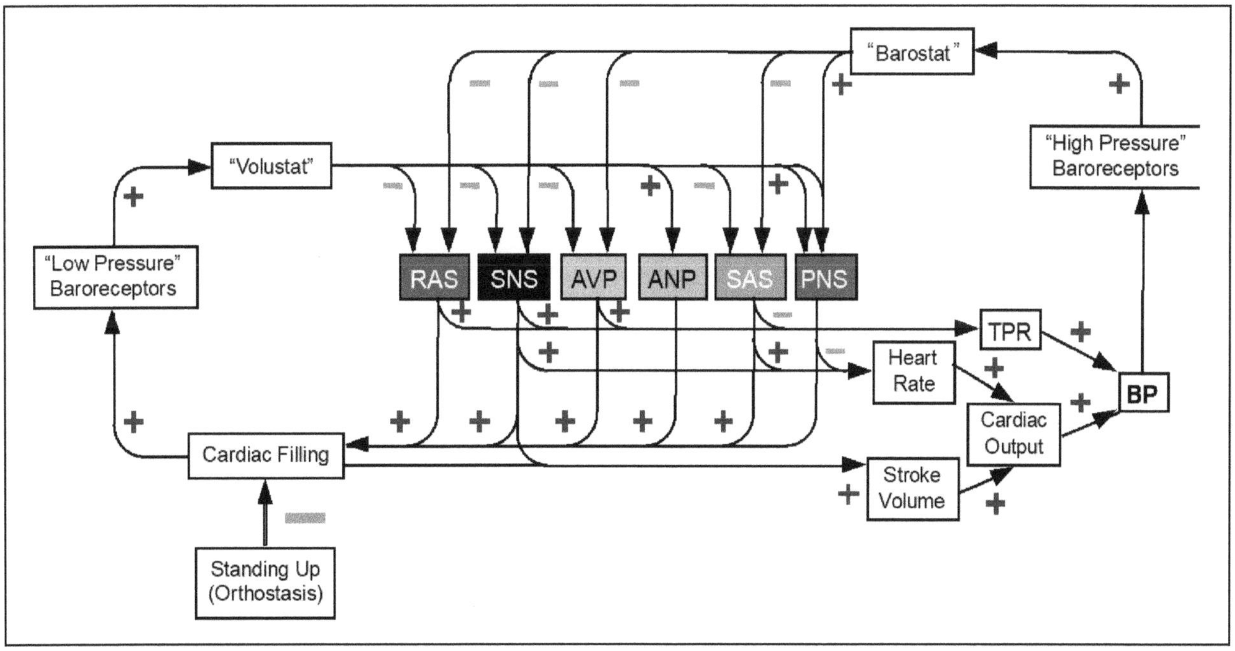

High pressure and low pressure barostatic systems use multiple effectors.

The "purpose" of the low-pressure baroreceptors is a guess, just as is the purpose of the high- pressure baroreceptors. In the schema shown in the concept diagram, the low-pressure baroreceptors are depicted as involved with regulation of extracellular fluid volume or blood volume; the corresponding homeostat is the "volustat."

A homeostatic definition of stress

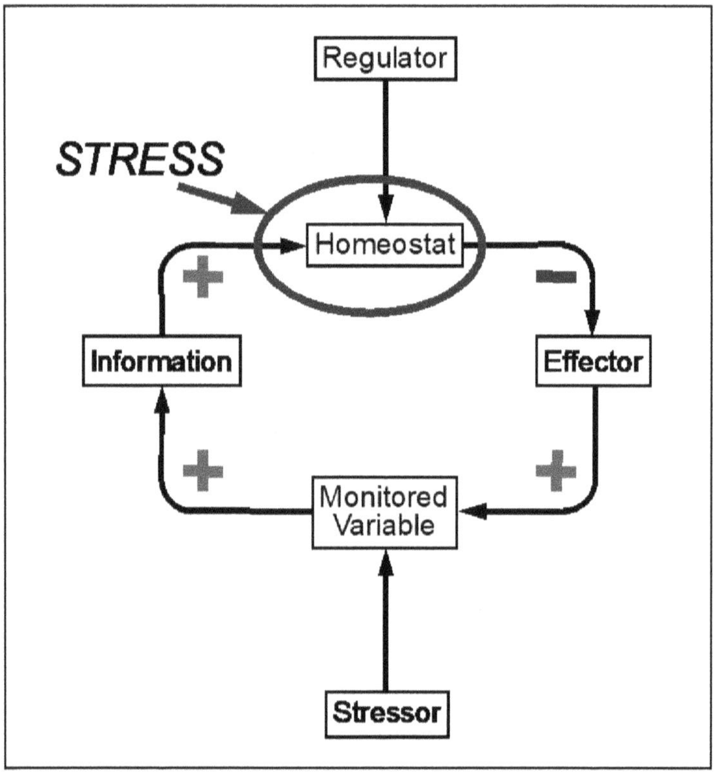

According to a homeostatic definition, stress is a condition in which the brain senses a discrepancy between information about the "inner world" and instructions for responding.

According to the homeostat theory, stress is neither a stimulus nor a stereotyped response pattern but a condition, a state in which there is a perceived discrepancy between information about the level of a monitored variable and an algorithm for responding, such that the discrepancy leads to alterations in activities of effectors—including components of the autonomic nervous system—closing a negative feedback loop and reducing the discrepancy.

Allostasis and allostatic load

Allostasis refers to a temporary shift in an input-output curve.

A low-grade fever when you have the flu is an example of allostasis. Anyone who has had a bad cold with a low-grade fever for a few days knows from personal experience what allostasis is. Your core temperature is higher, your pulse rate is faster, you lose your appetite, you curl up in bed, you sleep more, you withdraw socially, and you become cranky. You are "not yourself."

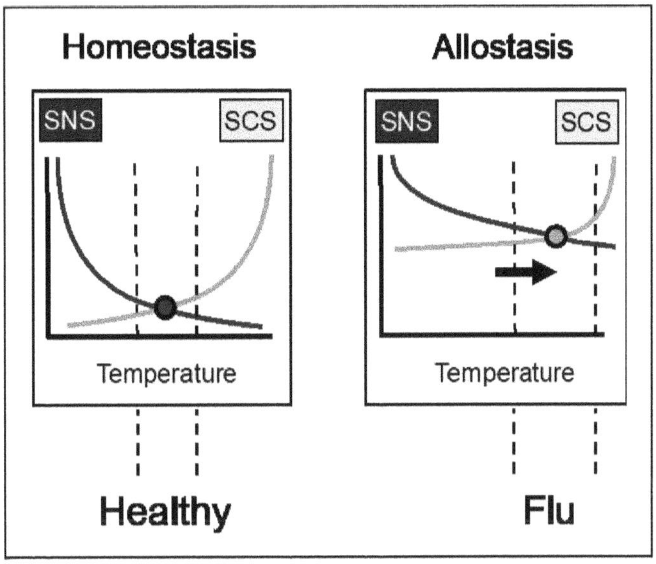

Shifts in input-output curves for the sympathetic noradrenergic system (SNS) and sympathetic cholinergic system exemplify allostatic adjustments.

When you have an acute illness like this, the levels of internal variables do not change in a completely uncontrolled way. Your core temperature is regulated but at a different thermostatic setting.

Allostatic adjustments use up more energy than do homeostatic adjustments. There is wear and tear on the effector systems— allostatic load. Allostatic load can decrease the efficiencies of the effectors, flattening the input-output curves. The decreased effector efficiencies increase the range of permitted levels of the monitored variable. Allostatic load corresponds to long-term wear and tear.

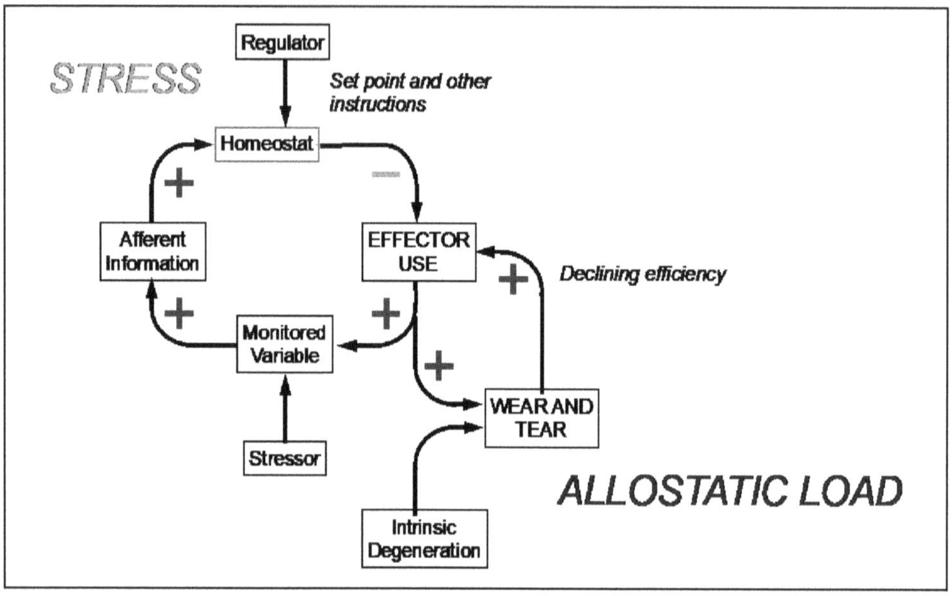

Homeostatic definitions of stress and allostatic load.

Allostatic load is like the wear and tear on your furnace as it cycles on and off during the winter. If you turned the thermostat way up, the furnace would be on more of the time, and there would be more wear and tear on its components.

If you not only turned the thermostat up but also left a large window open for the entire winter, there could be enough wear and tear on the furnace that it would fail completely.

Because of the wear and tear, the efficiency of the furnace declines. When the efficiency declines, then because of the negative feedback loop, the furnace is on more of the time. Because the furnace is on more of the time, there is more wear and tear, and the efficiency declines further.

This is an example of a positive feedback loop. The transition from a negative feedback loop to a positive feedback loop is a transition from a stable to an unstable internal environment and the end of homeostasis.

Wear and tear, combined with planned obsolescence, decreases effector efficiency. The same perturbation then results in greater wear and tear and further decreases effector efficiency. Eventually, even with the effectors activated maximally, the monitored variable drifts from the allostatic setting. Finally, when the effectors fail, the organism can no longer mount a stress response at all. This concept applies to the increased mortality of elderly persons when they are exposed to acute viral illnesses. As people age the efficiencies of their homeostatic systems decline. The ability to keep levels of monitored variables within healthy ranges is reduced. In the setting of this increased susceptibility, exposure to an acute stressor such as a viral illness is more likely to result in multi-organ failure and death.

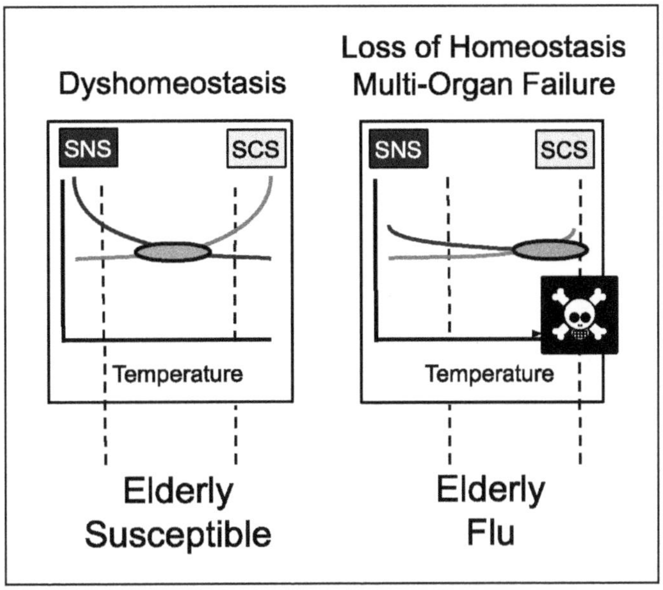

The homeostatic theory can explain why old people are at increased risk of dying from a viral illness.

Differential SNS & SAS responses to stressors

Walter B. Cannon conceptualized that the sympathoadrenal system functions as a unitary system maintaining homeostasis in emergencies. He taught that the body responds to all emergencies in the same way, by evoking increased secretion of adrenaline.

In fact, both the sympathetic noradrenergic system (SNS) and sympathetic adrenergic system (SAS) are active all the time.

Pulse-synchronous bursts of skeletal muscle SNS outflow and plasma levels of norepinephrine (NE) and adrenaline (epinephrine, EPI) are measurable in healthy people even during supine rest. There is no unitary sympathoadrenal response to all stressors.

Differential plasma EPI and NE responses across different stressors provide some of the strongest evidence that, in contrast with Cannon's view, there is no monolithic sympathoadrenal response to all stressors. The SAS is very sensitive to decreases in glucose availability, such as from insulin-induced hypoglycemia, and to emotional distress. Meanwhile, the SNS is very sensitive to cold exposure, isometric or mild exercise, active avoidance or escape behavior, and orthostasis (upright posture).

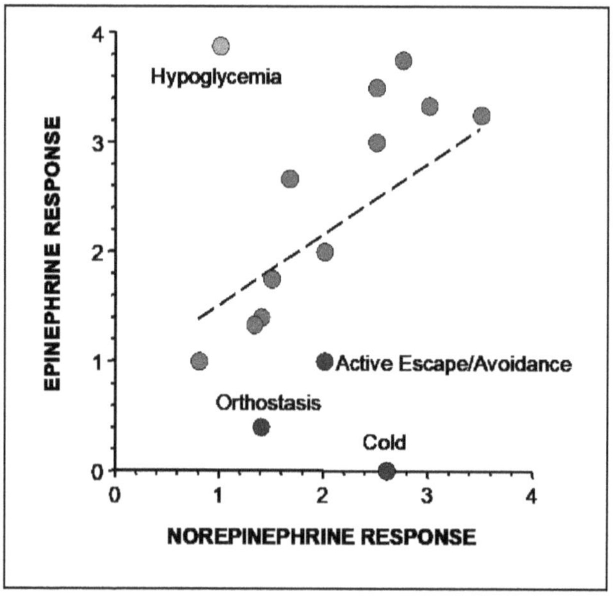

Differential responses of the sympathetic adrenergic system (SAS), for which epinephrine is the chemical messenger, and the sympathetic noradrenergic system (SNS), for which norepinephrine is the chemical messenger, argue against a monolithic sympathoadrenal system.

Across stressors plasma EPI responses actually are more closely tied to responses of the hypothalamic-pituitary- adrenocortical (HPA) axis, as indicated by corticotropin (ACTH) levels, than to responses of the SNS, as indicated by plasma NE levels. One can conceive of the existence of a unitary adrenal (adrenocortical/adrenomedullary) system just as easily as a unitary sympathoadrenal system.

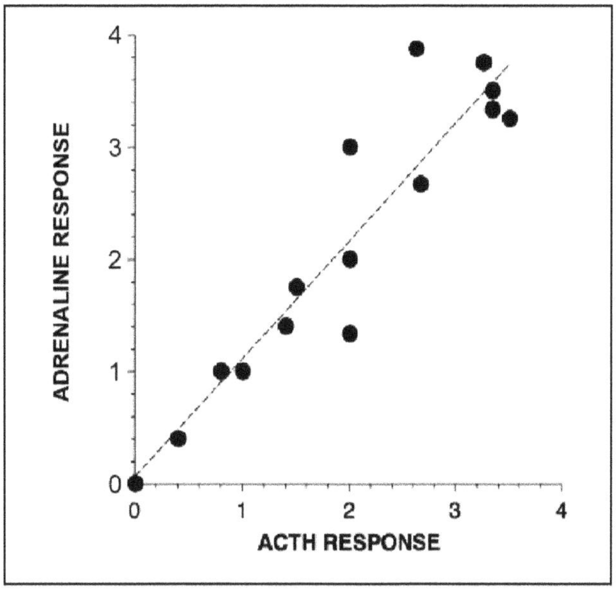

Across stressors there is a close association between the magnitude of the SAS response and the magnitude of response of the hypothalamic-pituitary-adrenocortical system as indicated by circulating corticotropin (ACTH).

Distress

Distress is a form of stress with additional characteristics—consciousness, aversiveness, observable signs, adrenal gland activation, and homeostatic resetting.

The experience of distress requires consciousness, because distress involves not only a challenge to homeostasis but also a perception by the organism that adjustments to meet that challenge may not suffice. Such perception implies an ability to interpret afferent nformation and to simulate future events, which in turn requires cerebral cortical activity.

Distress is negatively reinforcing and motivates escape and avoidance learning. Distressed organisms avoid situations that are perceived as likely to reproduce the same aversive experience.

The experience of distress enhances vigilance behavior and long-term memory of the distressing event. These adaptive adjustments probably offered substantial survival advantages in evolution. Bearing such an evolutionary history in mind helps understand potential long-term health consequences of distress such as in post-traumatic stress disorder (PTSD).

A third characteristic of distress is the evocation of signs that others can interpret as indicating the emotional state or intent of the organism. Perceptions of signs of distress by other members of the species automatically elicit involuntary, instinctive emotional and behavioral responses. The communication value of external signs of distress helps to explain the continued elaboration of observable components of distress responses in modern society, despite the relative rarity of true fight-or-flight reactions in humans. During the course of human evolution, these signs originally may have been by-products of genetically determined, autonomically mediated response patterns. In modern society, they continue to serve important signal functions.

Every hair follicle on your body has a small muscle called a pilomotor muscle, or arrector pili. When this muscle contracts the hair stands up. Coursing alongside the smooth muscle fibers are sympathetic noradrenergic nerves. Stimulation of the SNS causes the hair to bristle. The receptors on the smooth muscle cells are alpha-adrenoceptors. This means that circulating adrenaline, which is a universal adrenoceptor agonist, can also cause the hair to stand up.

Not only the sympathetic cholinergic system (SCS) but also the sympathetic noradrenergic system (SNS) and sympathetic adrenergic system (SAS) contribute to emotional sweating. Several years ago our nurse practitioner was going out for the evening and gave instructions to the babysitter. Her daughter had frequent asthma attacks, and so her mother wanted to demonstrate how to use an EpiPen™ in case there was an emergency. For practice she had a dummy pen, which could be reset by clicking the top—somewhat like clicking the top of a ball point pen. She showed the babysitter how easy it is to use an EpiPen™—just pull off the blue safety release and jab with the orange needle end against the outer thigh and hold it in place for about 10 seconds, to deliver the adrenaline. But when she jabbed herself, to her surprise she felt a sharp needle prick, which was odd for the blunt ended dummy pen; and when she pulled the pen from her thigh, she noticed that she couldn't reset the pen by clicking the top.

That was when she felt a wave of sweat spread over her body. Within several seconds her clothes were drenched. She also noticed she was hyperventilating and jittery and realized that instead of a dummy pen she had used a real EpiPen™ and had injected adrenaline into her leg.

During distress people turn pale. One way to understand this is that EPI potently constricts cutaneous blood vessels. At the same time and for the same reason that the skin becomes pale during distress, the skin also turns cold. When arterioles in the skin constrict, delivery of blood to the skin's surface decreases. Since the arteries carry blood to the skin at the core temperature, the temperature of the skin falls toward that of the cooler environment. You develop "cold feet" and break out in a "cold sweat."

Tremulousness is another instinctively communicated sign of fear to the point of panic that has been appreciated by writers since ancient times. To "shudder," "quiver," "quake," and "quail" not only mean to tremble but to do so in fear or uncertainty. Trembling and shivering during distress probably reflect activation of the SNS, since, as Cannon first showed, surgical inactivation of the adrenal glands augments rather than prevents shivering of animals exposed to cold. I have observed that during an infusion of yohimbine, which releases NE from sympathetic nerves, people can have such severe jaw trembling that their teeth chatter.

Musicians with stage fright or performance anxiety sometimes take a beta-adrenoceptor blocker before concerts. A friend of mine who is a professional cellist once told me that not only did several of his colleagues take a beta-blocker prophylactically before a concert but also that he could tell when they had done so. The performance would be technically accurate but with a subtle emotional restraint and detachment.

The gastrointestinal tract is also highly sensitive to distress. Recall that Walter B. Cannon's initial demonstration of EPI release during distress was based on the blood of the "excited" animal inhibiting spontaneously contractions of an intestinal strip of tissue.

We all know that emotion-related feats of strength and speed are associated with remarkable loss of the sensation of pain. This is called "stress-induced analgesia." Adrenaline or norepinephrine may alter the experience of pain by occupying alpha-2 adrenoceptors in the spinal cord. These receptors appear to contribute to a "gate" for transmitting pain impulses up to the brain. The source of the chemical transmitter that would occupy these alpha-2 adrenoceptors may not be circulating adrenaline, or even norepinephrine released as a neurotransmitter from sympathetic nerves, but norepinephrine released from nerves that project from the brainstem to the spinal cord. The locus ceruleus, a small cluster of cells in the back of the pons, is the main source of norepinephrine in the brain. Locus ceruleus neurons send widely branching fibers throughout the brain, probably contributing to psycho-emotional phenomena such as vigilance and the memory of distressing events. It is unclear whether locus ceruleus neurons are the source of the norepinephrine that modulates the transmission of pain impulses in the spinal cord. The main known modulators of pain sensation are endogenous opioids. Behaviors such as exercise increase occupation of opioid receptors in the brain, explaining the sense of elation some people feel after a workout. In response to painful stimuli, the brain releases opioids that apparently limit the severity of experienced pain, because blockade of opioid receptors augments the amount of pain for a given amount of stimulation. Blockade of opioid receptors also augments the release of EPI. Finally, stimulation of the adrenal gland releases not only EPI but also endogenous painkiller opiates called enkephalins.

Another characteristic of distress is adrenal gland activation. This involves enhanced release of catecholamines from the adrenal medulla and of glucocorticoids from the adrenal cortex. As noted above, EPI seems to be a key determinant of communicated signs of distress.

Although Cannon viewed the neural and hormonal components of the "sympathico-adrenal" system as functioning as a unit to preserve homeostasis in emergencies, a more modern view holds that it is specifically the adrenomedullary hormonal component that characterizes distress, while SNS outflows may increase, decrease, or stay the same. This might depend partly on whether there is a locomotor response (e.g., escape behavior), which entails increased skeletal muscle sympathetic noradrenergic outflows as part of "central command." Plasma levels of adrenaline constitute an extraordinarily rapid and sensitive chemical index of this activation and therefore of experienced distress.

A final characteristic of distress is that it is associated with shifts in input-output curves determining autonomic outflows. These in essence are allostatic changes. An example is the shift in arterial baroreflex function curves during distress.

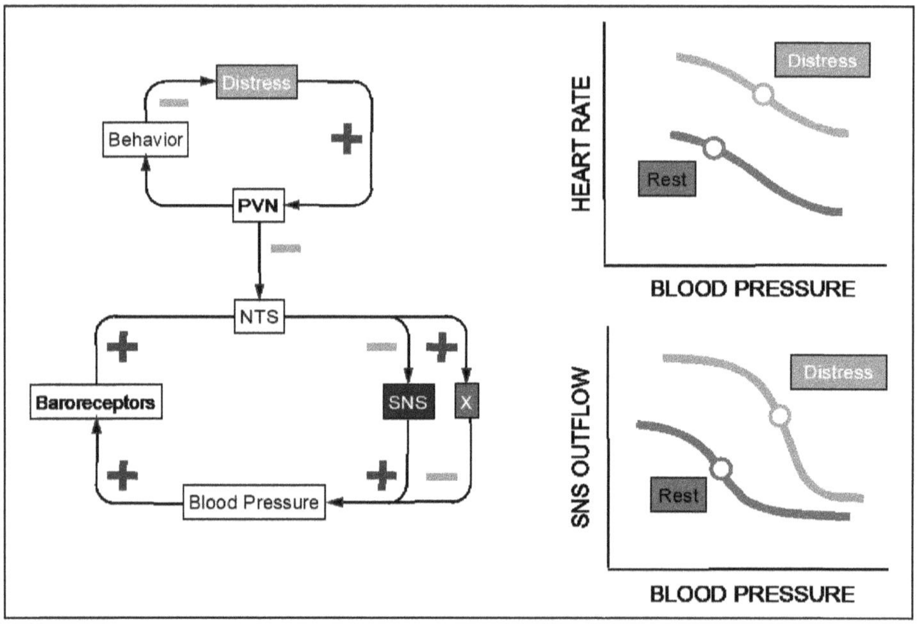

Distress shifts barostatic input-output curves—an example of allostasis.

Adaptation and resilience

Higher organisms have capabilities to habituate, anticipate, heal, regenerate, and in general increase resilience. These processes may operate at multiple sites within homeostatic loops to increase the useful life of the effectors for the same amount of chronic exposure to a stressor.

One can conceive of a non-circular definition of eustress that is a kind of mirror image of the non-circular definition of distress. Just as distress is consciously experienced, negatively reinforcing, motivates escape and avoidance behavior, and enhances vigilance, eustress is consciously experienced, positively reinforcing, motivates approach and appetitive behavior, and enhances attention to oneself. Both distress and eustress have offered survival advantages in evolution, but either can be pathogenic in the setting of modern humanity.

That is, neither may be only good or only bad for health. Just as modern-day pathologic consequences of distress are thought to include panic/anxiety, melancholic depression, or post- traumatic stress disorder, pathologic consequences of eustress might include drug and alcohol abuse, sex offenses, gambling and other risk-taking behaviors, and overeating.

Organisms can protect and repair themselves after stress and even learn to anticipate and proactively make "feed-forward" adjustments that mitigate damage from future stress exposures. The concept is emerging that certain aspects of lifestyle, such as exercise training and some psychological interventions, enhance resilience. There is evidence that repeated exposures may increase resilience to heterotypic stressors.

AUTONOMIC FUNCTION TESTS

Symptoms and signs of dysautonomias result from alterations in activities of one or more components of the ANS. Particular autonomic abnormalities manifest clinically in symptoms or signs that may give clues about inhibition or activation of a particular component of the ANS.

Sympathetic noradrenergic system (SNS) activation

Increased activity of the sympathetic noradrenergic system (SNS) produces its effects via the release of norepinephrine (NE).

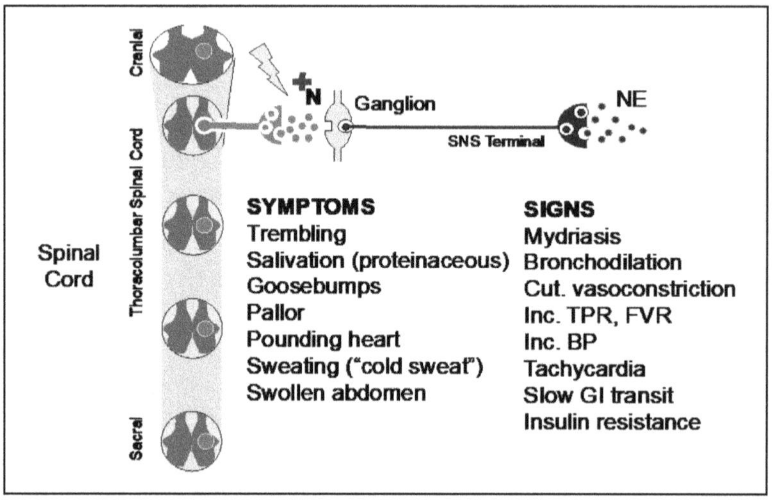

Symptoms and signs of generalized SNS activation.

The released NE constricts blood vessels in the skin, kidneys, gut, and skeletal muscle. Because of the constriction of blood vessels in the skin the patient may look pale.

NE released from sympathetic nerves in the skin also causes the hair to stand up and produces goosebumps. Stimulation of the sympathetic nerves in the salivary glands increases the flow of thick saliva. Other manifestations of increased SNS outflows include increased blood pressure or heart rate, pallor, and trembling. Gastrointestinal functions are inhibited.

SNS inhibition

Conversely, SNS failure typically manifests as orthostatic hypotension (OH). SNS failure can also produce low blood pressure after eating a meal post-prandial hypotension), after exercising, or upon exposure to warm temperature.

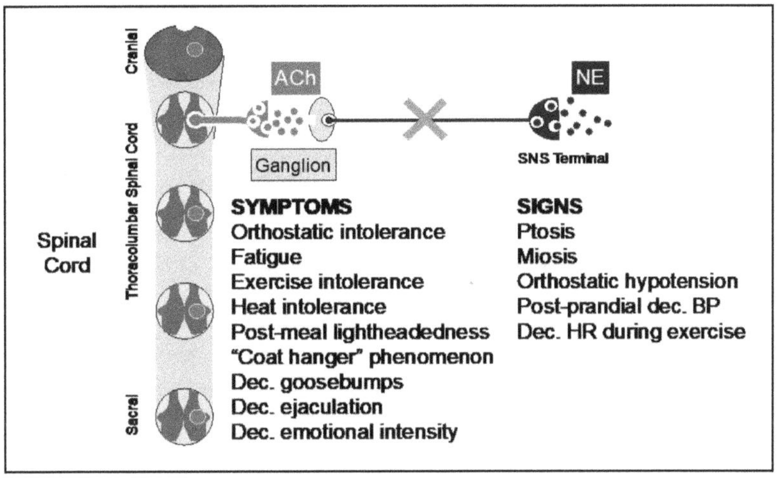

Symptoms and signs of SNS inhibition or failure.

SNS failure is also associated with a tendency to have less than the normal increase in the force and rate of the heartbeat during exercise. This could manifest clinically as fatigue, shortness of breath with exercise, or exercise intolerance.

A cardinal sign of SNS failure is OH.

Parasympathetic nervous system (PNS) activation

Increased activity of the parasympathetic nervous system (PNS) produces effects via release of acetylcholine in several organs of the body.

The patient notes increased gut motions, nausea, urinary urgency or frequency, increased production of watery saliva, increased tear production, and decreased visual adaptation

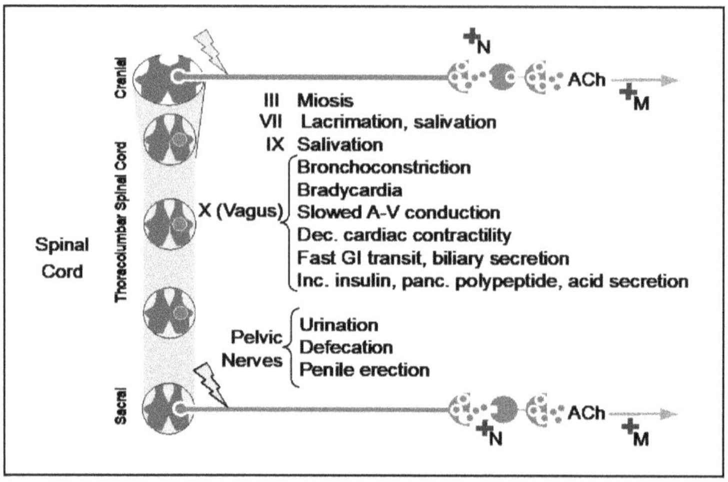

Effects of generalized parasympathetic nervous system activation.

in the dark. Signs of increased PNS activity include slowed heart rate, increased bowel sounds, increased salivation, increased tear production, and constricted pupils.

PNS inhibition

Parasympathetic nervous system (PNS) underactivity produces many symptoms, including dry mouth, constipation, urinary problems, decreased tear production, and (in men) inability to have an erection.

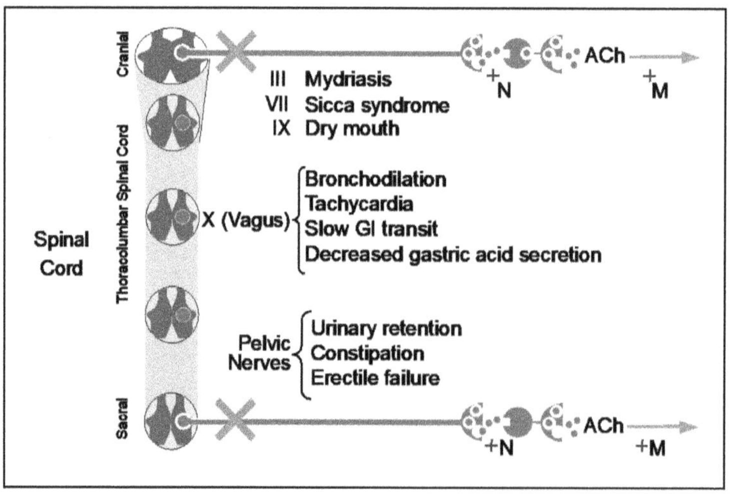

Effects of generalized parasympathetic nervous system inhibition or failure.

When the PNS is underactive, the person has a dry mouth (associated with a raspy voice), constipation, a tendency to retain urine in the bladder, a relatively fast pulse rate, dry eyes, and, in men, erectile failure. Several drugs can cause these symptoms, such as medications to treat urinary incontinence or diarrhea. Signs of PNS failure include decreased bowel sounds, increased heart rate, and enlargement of the urinary bladder due to urinary retention.

Sympathetic cholinergic system (SCS) activation

Increased activity of the sympathetic cholinergic system (SCS) produces effects via release of acetylcholine in sweat glands. The patient reports increased sweating—during heat exposure, exercise, after eating (gustatory sweating), during emotional distress, or at rest.

When the PNS is underactive, the person has a dry mouth (associated with a raspy voice), constipation, a tendency to retain urine in the bladder, a relatively fast pulse rate, dry eyes, and, in men, erectile failure. Several drugs can cause these symptoms, such as medications to treat urinary incontinence or diarrhea. Signs of PNS failure include decreased bowel sounds, increased heart rate, and enlargement of the urinary bladder due to urinary retention.

Increased activity of the sympathetic cholinergic system (SCS) produces effects via release of acetylcholine in sweat glands. The patient reports increased sweating—during heat exposure, exercise, after eating (gustatory sweating), during emotional distress, or at rest.

SCS inhibition

The symptoms and signs of SCS failure are from decreased sweating. Since acetylcholine is the main chemical messenger used by the sympathetic nervous system for sweating, NE is the main chemical messenger used by the sympathetic nervous system to tighten blood vessels and maintain blood pressure during standing. A patient with a specific problem in the production, release, or receptors for NE may have orthostatic hypotension and yet sweat normally.

Sympathetic adrenergic system (SAS) activation

Increased activity of the sympathetic adrenergic system (SAS) produces effects via release of epinephrine (EPI) from the adrenal glands.

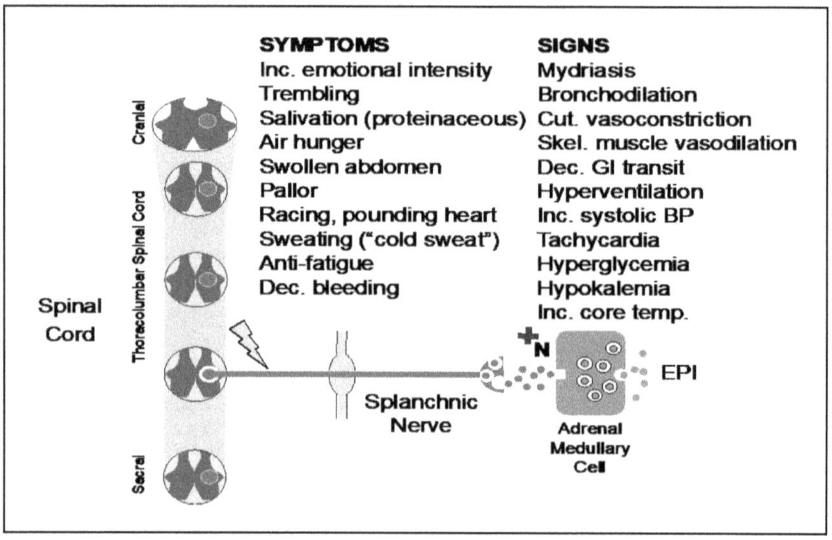

Symptoms and signs of SAS activation.

Symptoms of SAS activation may include a sense of energy or increased emotional intensity, anxiety, a sense of the heart beating (palpitation), an increased rate or depth of breathing, and abdominal bloating, pain, or nausea. Signs of SAS activation include pallor of the skin (due to constriction of cutaneous blood vessels), trembling, a tendency toward decreased bleeding time (due to platelet activation), sweating, and increased blood glucose levels.

SAS inhibition

Whether SAS failure produces symptoms or signs is unclear. Perhaps there is a tendency to hypoglycemia or decreased emotional intensity.

The Most Important Autonomic Function Test

Symptoms are feelings that the patient reports to the medical professional as part of the medical history. Signs are medical findings that a medical professional detects during a physical examination.

The autonomic medical history

The most important autonomic function test is the medical history, which consists of several parts. These include the Chief Complaint, the History of the Present Illness (HPI), the Past History, the Family History, the Personal and Social History, and the Review of Systems (ROS). Each of these parts is important for diagnosing and managing dysautonomias, but of these the key components are the Chief Complaint and the HPI.

The Chief Complaint is a single phrase or sentence that describes in the patients' own words what has been bothering them that has led to the evaluation.

Chief Complaint: In a few words, what's the main problem bothering you that brings you here today?

HPI: When was the last time you felt completely healthy?
What was the first thing that went wrong?
What happened next?
Have you noticed anything that makes the problem worse or better?
What treatments have been tried, and how did you respond?

Autonomic ROS:
Who does your shopping? Are you able to tolerate standing, exercise, heat, a large meal?
Do you sweat like other people?
Do you make spit like other people?
Have you noticed any problems with urination?
Have you noticed any problems with bowel movements?
Have you noticed any problems with sexual function?

Components of the autonomic medical history.

The chief complaint

The chief complaint, despite being only a phrase or sentence, can be remarkably informative. I once evaluated a local elderly woman who was referred for pure autonomic failure, because she had persistent, consistent orthostatic hypotension. I asked her, "We'll be going into detail about your medical history, but for now, in a single phrase or sentence, can you tell me what it is that's been bothering you that's brought you here today?" I was expecting she would report dizziness or lightheadedness when she was upright, or perhaps fainting episodes while standing in line at a checkout counter. Instead, her chief complaint was that she couldn't make spit and she was constipated.

Dry mouth and constipation are symptoms of parasympathetic nervous system (PNS) failure, not sympathetic noradrenergic system (SNS) failure. I asked if she sweated like other people, and she said no, because she couldn't sweat at all. Sweating is a sympathetic cholinergic system (SCS) function. In other words, she had symptoms of a pandysautonomia that involved failure of all the components of the autonomic nervous system.

Eventually she was found not to have pure autonomic failure but a previously undescribed condition, autoimmune autonomic ganglionopathy from a circulating antibody to the neuronal nicotinic receptor. The initial clue to the diagnosis was her unexpected chief complaint.

The history of the present illness (HPI)

The HPI is a narrative history of the condition. It is best to obtain the HPI from the patient directly. Of course there are records to review of hospitalizations, test results, previous accounts of the medical history, and physical examination; however, these are subject to mistakes and often are uninformative. On the other hand, the patient's own story of the chronology of his or her symptoms, especially with the help of family or significant others, is likely to be both correct and informative.

Obtaining the medical history, especially the HPI, is a skill that must be honed by learning and experience, ideally under the supervision of a mentor.

Medications

A complete listing of all prescribed and over-the-counter medications, herbal remedies, and dietary supplements is a key part of the medical history, not only because these agents can affect autonomic functions and complicate or confound test results but also because they can interact with each other or with the condition to produce unanticipated problems and serious adverse events.

Even herbal remedies must be considered carefully. Years ago I had a patient with multiple system atrophy (MSA) who first came to medical attention because of paroxysmal high blood pressure after taking ma huang tea. He had thought this would alleviate his sense of fatigue and lack of energy. The active ingredient in ma huang is ephedrine, an amphetamine. The drug increased delivery of NE to its receptors, which caused the blood pressure to increase, and because of baroreflex failure, which is part of the clinical laboratory picture in MSA, the increase in blood pressure was not buffered by the baroreflex. The patient developed a severe headache and went to the emergency room. Because of his headache and paroxysmal hypertension the physicians thought at first that he was having a stroke from subarachnoid hemorrhage.

Ma huang is no longer sold as a dietary supplement in the US, but yohimbe bark is. Yohimbine, a drug derived from yohimbe bark, increases norepinephrine release. In a patient with baroreflex failure, taking this NE supplement could result in severe hypertension, just as in the MSA patient.

Timing is everything

In obtaining the history of the present illness (HPI) one of the most important skills a clinician can acquire is the ability to get the sequence straight. I usually start by asking the patient, "When was the last time you felt completely well?" The answer can range from "I've always been sick," to "I was fine until…" a particular date, to "It was such a gradual thing, I don't know."

Some dysautonomias develop in a rather stereotyped sequence. An example is the cerebellar form of multiple system atrophy (MSA-C) in a man. Men with MSA-C typically relate that the first thing to go wrong, in retrospect, was erectile failure. In my opinion, in a man with central neurodegeneration and orthostatic hypotension, the absence of erectile failure as an early finding rules out MSA-C. The erectile failure is followed by urinary problems—especially urinary retention, eventually to the point of requiring self-catheterization. Then come slurred speech, a wide-based, unsteady gait "like a drunken sailor," and lightheadedness when standing.

In obtaining the details about symptoms of dysautonomias, it is also important to determine which situations make things worse and which make them better. For instance, patients with neurogenic orthostatic hypotension often relate that their symptoms are worst in the morning, upon heat exposure, after eating a large meal, or after exercise.

Because of associations of autonomic failure with non-motor aspects of Parkinson's disease and other Lewy body diseases, it is important to ask about whether the patient is able to smell things like other people do, whether the patient sees things like other people do, and whether the patient has any problems with sleep. The clinician is looking for evidence of olfactory dysfunction, visual hallucinations (a feature suggestive of dementia with Lewy bodies), and dream enactment behavior.

In patients with possible postural tachycardia syndrome (POTS) it is valuable to ask about whether the patient has "double-jointedness" or stretchy skin, since these can be clues to the occurrence of Ehlers-Danlos syndrome. Later on you will learn about the "coat hanger sign" and the "water bottle sign" in dysautonomias like POTS.

Again, the sequence of events can be very informative. Subacute development of orthostatic intolerance after a viral illness suggests an autoimmune pathophysiology, whereas a history since childhood of frequent fainting or "seizures" suggests a congenital, genetic component. In the evaluation of a patient with POTS, which occurs mainly in relatively young women, it is important to ask, in a private setting, about emotional, physical, or sexual abuse in childhood. These can have long-term consequences in terms of chronic fatigue, altered memory or concentration, post-traumatic stress disorder, and panic or anxiety.

In a patient with labile blood pressure and orthostatic intolerance, a remote history of irradiation of the neck brings up the possibility of arterial baroreflex failure due to accelerated arteriosclerosis in the carotid sinus area.

My screening questions generally query each of the components of the autonomic nervous system. The questions are designed not to be leading. For instance, about sympathetic cholinergic function, I ask, "Do you sweat like other people?" About sympathetic noradrenergic function, I ask, "Do you have any issues standing still?" About parasympathetic cholinergic function, I ask, "Are you able to make spit and tears like other people?" Have you noticed anything different about how your GI system is working? Have you noticed anything different about your urination? In a man I ask, "Are you able to have an erection and ejaculate?"

A pain in the neck

In patients with orthostatic intolerance or orthostatic hypotension, standing upright can result in an annoying pain in the back of the neck and along the shoulders. Because of the distribution of the discomfort, this is sometimes referred to as coat hanger pain.

"Coat hanger" pain can be brought on by orthostasis.

The mechanism of the coat hanger phenomenon is not well understood. I think of it as a kind of cramp, when the anti- gravity muscles holding up the head receive too little blood flow. These muscles are active all the time, which means that they are continuously using up the oxygen that is delivered to them via the arterial blood. If the blood flow falls to below a certain rate, then metabolic waste products can build up that produce pain.

Who does your shopping?

Most patients with chronic orthostatic intolerance are women. At the risk of seeming chauvinistic, a screening question I ask to a woman referred for orthostatic intolerance is, "Who does your shopping?" A positive answer is something like, "Well not me. I can't tolerate standing still in line. I start to feel faint or lightheaded or weak, or I have to sit down, or I have to twist my legs like a pretzel."

Pretzel legs

I remember well the first patient I ever saw with pure autonomic failure (PAF). PAF is a rare disease in which orthostatic hypotension dominates the clinical picture. She was sitting in a chair in the examining room with her legs twisted around each other like a pretzel. She had learned from experience that doing this when she was sitting up delayed the onset of lightheadedness. By working the muscles of the legs against each other and tightening her buttocks she was squeezing blood upward in her body toward the heart.

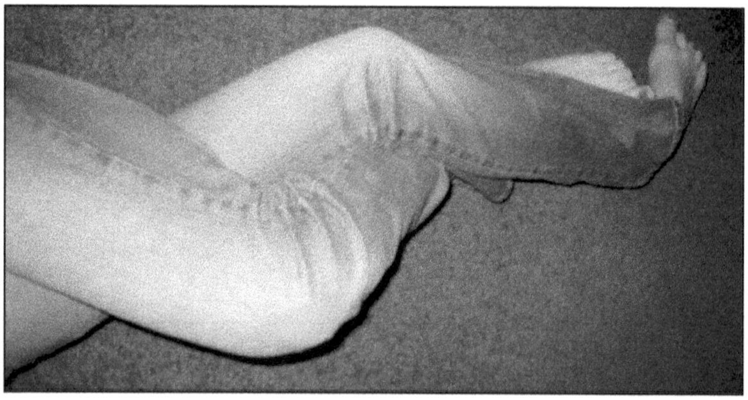

"Pretzel legs" is a common finding in chronic orthostatic intolerance.

When there is deficient reflexive sympathetically-mediated vasoconstriction during orthostasis, "pretzel legs" help maintain venous return to the heart. Adopting this posture can be an effective countermeasure in patients with autonomically mediated presyncope.

Water bottle sign

It is common for a patient with orthostatic intolerance to bring a bottle of water to the clinical encounter and sip from it periodically as the history is taken. I call this the "water bottle sign." The patients often report that although drinking water doesn't eliminate the symptoms, not drinking water rapidly makes them worse.

To me this could be a clue as to the pathophysiology of chronic orthostatic intolerance. Perhaps the kidneys are less efficient in reabsorbing filtered water, and the water bottle sign is part of a behavioral compensation. The kidneys filter about 100 mL of plasma per minute, or about 144 liters per day. Since normal urine output is about 1.5 liters per day, the kidneys are roughly 99% efficient in reabsorbing water. One might expect that even the slightest decrease in the efficiency of water reabsorption would result in a tendency to dehydration.

A bit of a stretch

Joint hypermobility ("double jointedness") occurs rather frequently among patients with postural tachycardia syndrome (POTS). When obtaining the medical history in a patient with chronic orthostatic intolerance, it is worthwhile to ask whether the patient is double jointed and if so to ask what sorts of "tricks" the patient can perform with his/her body that other people can't.

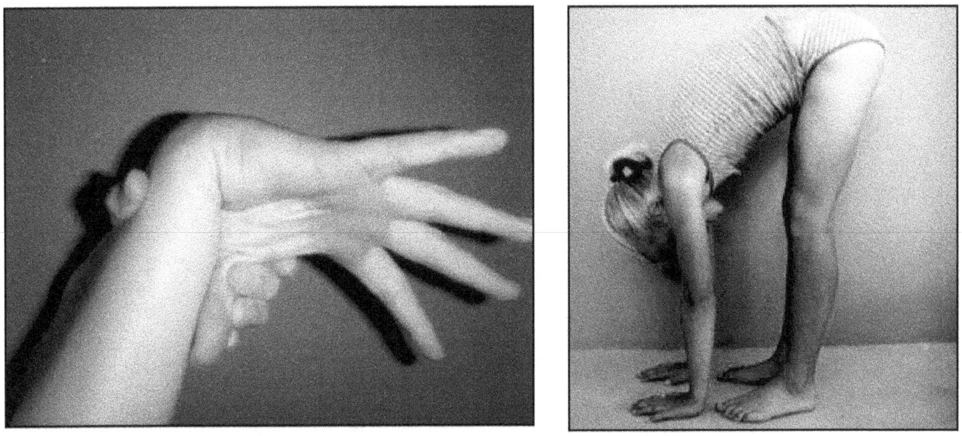

Two signs of joint hypermobility.

Ehlers-Danlos syndrome (EDS) is an inherited connective tissue disease in which the patients have joint hypermobility, lax skin, a tendency to joint dislocation or subluxation, musculoskeletal pain, and easy bruising. EDS patients often have a "Marfanoid" appearance, in that they are tall, thin, have long arms and legs, and have long thin fingers (arachnodactyly, or "spider fingers"), as in the Marfan syndrome. POTS occurs frequently in EDS, for reasons that remain poorly understood. A possible explanation for the association is that a problem with collagen in blood vessel walls makes them more stretchy or compliant, so that blood tends to pool in the abdomen or pelvis during standing.

Beighton scoring is used to gauge the severity of joint hypermobility, based on 5 tests. The Beighton score is calculated as follows:

1. One point for each little finger that you can bend backwards by more than 90 degrees.

2. One point for each thumb that you can touch to your forearm when bent backwards.
3. One point for each elbow that you can bend backwards.
4. One point for each knee that you can bend backwards.
5. One point if while standing you can bend forward and place your palms on the ground with your legs straight.

Florida Chinese restaurant syndrome

Orthostatic hypotension often is accompanied by post-prandial lightheadedness and hypotension. "Post-prandial" means after eating a meal. In patients with SNS failure, heat exposure also can decrease the blood pressure.

I refer to this combination as "Florida Chinese Restaurant Syndrome." Picture a stereotypical elderly male retiree in Florida who happens to have SNS failure. He visits an all-you- can-eat Chinese buffet restaurant, which is air conditioned and chilly if not downright cold inside. Over the course of about a half hour he stuffs himself with food, and then he leaves. Meanwhile, his car has been baking in the sun in the parking lot, and it is blistering hot when he gets in. A few minutes later he enters the local lanes on the way to I-95, sitting upright at the wheel and almost motionless. Soon after accelerating to get into the express lanes of I-95 at high speed, he begins to feel lightheaded; his limbs don't work, and he can't think straight. He loses control of the car and is injured or killed in an accident. The take-home point is that in patients with failure of the sympathetic noradrenergic system (SNS), post-prandial hypotension, cutaneous vasodilation from intense heat exposure, orthostatic hypotension, and absence of muscle pumping constitute a highly morbid and potentially lethal combination.

Physiological tests

Physiological autonomic function tests involve measurements taken in response to a manipulation such as deep breathing, standing, tilt table-testing, or a change in room temperature.

There are always several steps between the brain's directing changes in nerve traffic in the autonomic nervous system and the physiological measures that are chosen to track the autonomic changes. Because of this indirectness, results of physiological tests can be difficult to interpret or may not identify a problem accurately.

Orthostatic vital signs

Measuring the blood pressure (BP) during supine rest and then after being upright is required to identify orthostatic hypotension (OH), which in turn is a key manifestation of failure of the sympathetic noradrenergic system.

According to a consensus of autonomics experts, OH is "a sustained reduction of systolic blood pressure of at least 20 mmHg or diastolic blood pressure of 10 mmHg within 3 min of standing or head-up tilt to at least 60° on a tilt table."

In my opinion, before the baseline BP is measured, the patient should be supine (with head on pillow) for at least 10 minutes. During this time, the observer can list all the medications and dietary supplements that the patient has taken within the past 24 hours and when they were taken. The location of the measurement, the time of day, and when and what the patient last ate should be noted (the latter because of the possibility of post-prandial hypotension).

In order to avoid gravitational effects when the brachial cuff is below heart level, the patient's arm should be supported at heart level when the patient is upright. The patient should not have the arm extended without support, because this introduces the possibility of effects of isometric exercise on the measurement.

Heart rate usually is measured simultaneously with BP. Patients with baroreflex-cardiovagal failure have a small orthostatic increment in heart rate for a given fall in BP; however, such patients still have some increase in heart rate. The occurrence of an increase in heart rate during standing should not be taken as evidence against neurogenic OH.

Heart rate variability

When you take in a slow, deep breath, your pulse rate increases, and when you then breathe out, your pulse rate falls. The wave- like rhythmic change in the heart rate due to breathing is called respiratory sinus arrhythmia. Despite the word, arrhythmia, meaning "lacking rhythm," respiratory sinus arrhythmia is quite rhythmic and quite normal. The Dutch cardiologist Karel Frederik Wenckebach wrote in the early 1900s that a variable pulse rate is the sign of a healthy heart. These changes result mainly from modulation of parasympathetic nervous system (PNS) outflow to the heart via the vagus nerve.

If you recorded the cardiac interbeat interval across many heartbeats and graphed the number of beats in bins of interbeat intervals, you would see a bell-shaped curve, as in the diagram. The more variable the heart rate, the wider the bell-shaped curve. This is called analysis of heart rate variability in the time domain.

With aging, heart failure, and most forms of chronic autonomic failure, the heart rate becomes more stable. The bell-shaped curve becomes narrower. This is probably not from altered autonomic innervation of the heart but from decreased reflexive modulation of traffic in nerves supplying the heart.

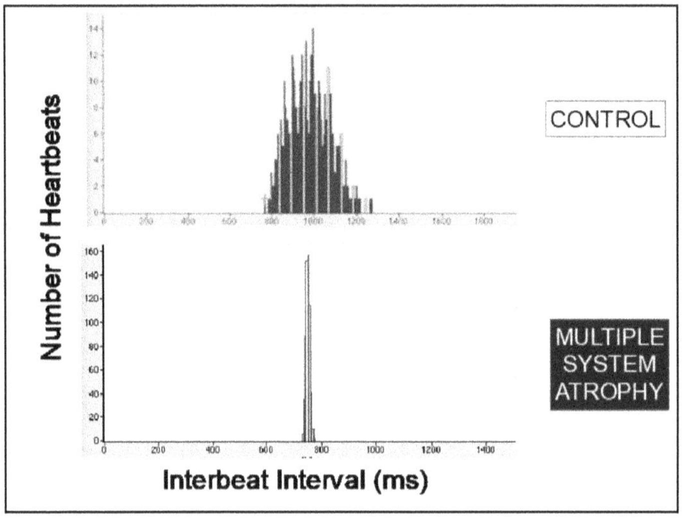

Heart rate variability in the time domain. Baroreflex-cardiovagal failure is common in multiple system atrophy.

Heart rate variability can also be assessed in the frequency domain.

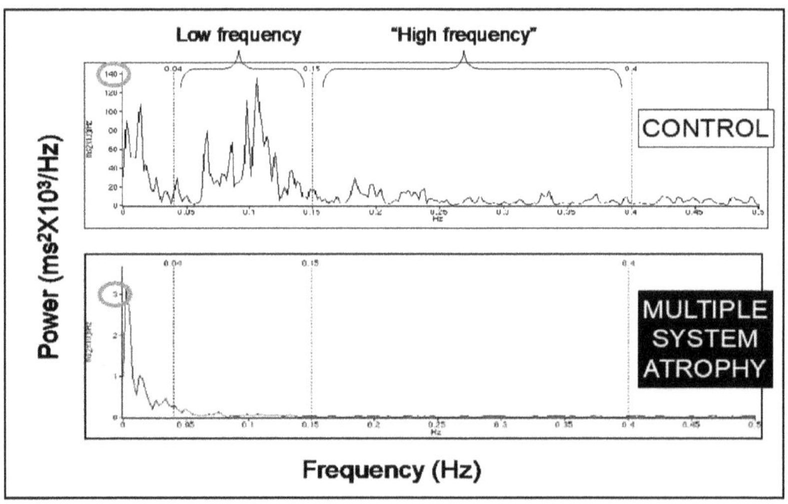

Heart rate variability in the frequency domain.

High frequency power (at the frequency of respiration) is a measure of respiratory sinus arrhythmia and therefore of baroreflex-cardiovagal function. Low frequency power has been thought to at least partly reflect cardiac sympathetic "tone" but probably more likely reflects the ability to modulate cardiac sympathetic tone via baroreflexes.

The Valsalva maneuver

The Valsalva maneuver test is one of the most important clinical physiological tests for autonomic failure. The test is done using a method to measure blood pressure continuously (beat-to-beat). The maneuver consists of blowing against a resistance for several seconds and then relaxing.

The patient may be asked to blow into a tube connected to a blood pressure gauge, moving the gauge's needle to a particular pressure (30-40 mmHg) and keeping the needle there for 10-15 seconds.

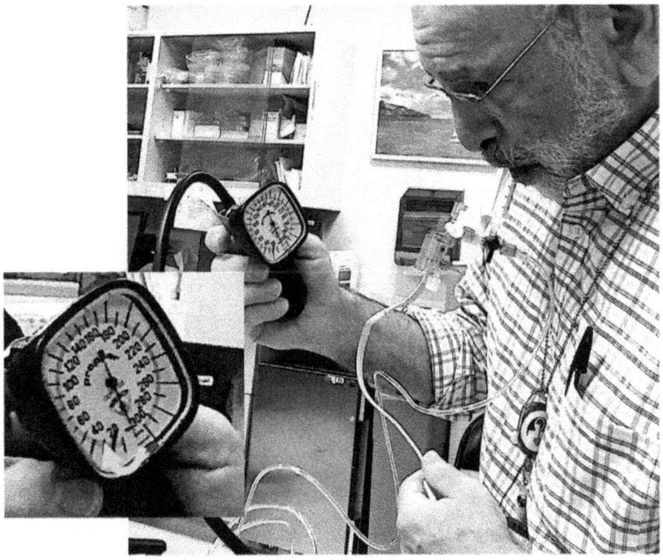

In the Valsalva maneuver one blows against a resistance for several seconds and then relaxes.

In Phase I, just after starting to squeeze, the blood is forced out of the chest, and the blood pressure increases briefly. This is mechanical and has nothing to do with reflexes.

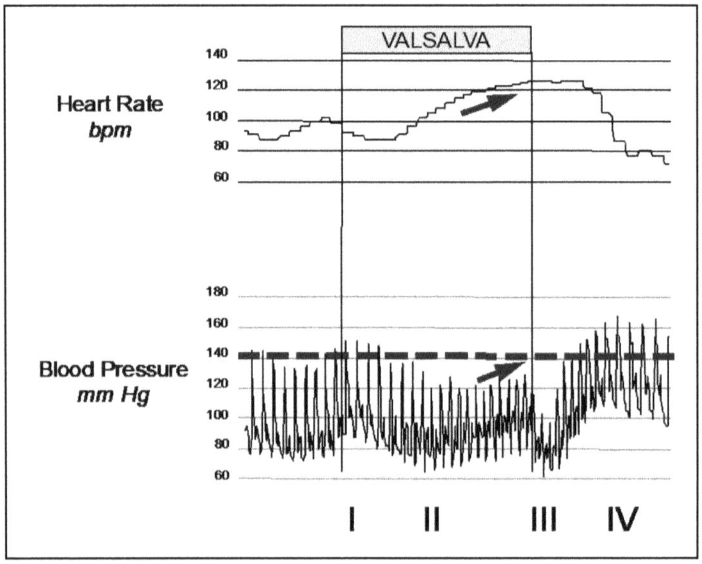

Normal responses to the Valsalva maneuver.

As you continue to strain, the high pressure in the chest and abdomen results in less blood reaching the heart, and the heart pumps less blood, so normally in Phase II the blood pressure falls. The brain picks up on this immediately and directs a reflex to occur in which outflows in the sympathetic noradrenergic system (SNS) increase, norepinephrine, the chemical messenger of the SNS, is released, the norepinephrine binds to its receptors in the heart and blood vessel walls, and the blood vessels constrict. As a result, at the end of Phase II blood pressure increases, even though the heart is still pumping out less blood. Also during Phase II the heart rate normally goes up, due to withdrawal of parasympathetic nervous system outflow to the heart via the vagus nerve.

Then the patient relaxes. The blood pressure immediately falls (Phase III)—a kind of mirror image of the increase in Phase I. The decrease in pressure in Phase III has nothing to do with reflexes. Finally, in Phase IV the patient is relaxed, and now there is no impediment in blood returning to the heart. The heart pumps the blood, but it pumps the blood into the reflexively constricted vasculature, and so the blood pressure rapidly increases and overshoots the baseline value.

In a patient with failure of this reflex—whether because of a decrease in afferent information from the baroreceptors to the brain, or because the brain doesn't act on the information due a brain disease, or because the sympathetic nerves are gone, or because norepinephrine isn't released, or because the adrenoceptors receptors are blocked—there is the same abnormal pattern of blood pressure (BP) during and after the Valsalva maneuver. In Phase II the BP goes down progressively, because the patient can't tighten the vascular nozzle, and in Phase IV the BP returns slowly to the baseline value but doesn't overshoot the baseline value, for the same reason. These are signs of baroreflex-sympathoneural failure.

In most (but not all) forms of chronic autonomic failure manifesting with orthostatic hypotension, the heart rate doesn't change as much as it should given the magnitude of the fall in blood pressure. The extent of increase in heart rate (or more formally the extent of decrease in the cardiac interbeat interval) per mmHg decrease in systolic blood pressure during Phase II of the Valsalva maneuver is a measure of baroreflex-cardiovagal gain.

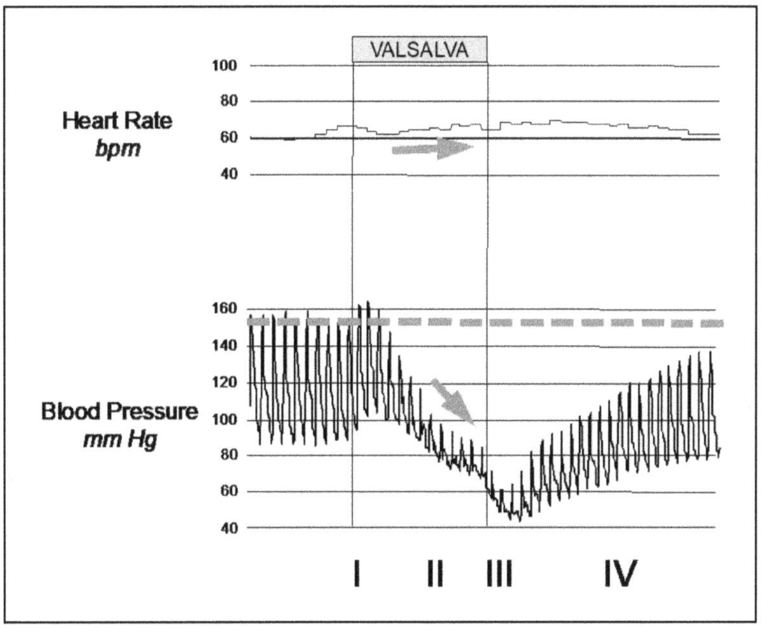

Baroreflex-sympathoneural and baroreflex-cardiovagal failure detected by continuous blood pressure and heart rate responses to the Valsalva maneuver.

Note that one must monitor the blood pressure (BP) changes beat-to-beat in order to identify baroreflex-sympathoneural failure based on the BP responses to the Valsalva maneuver. Until recently such continuous monitoring required insertion of a catheter into an artery. Since physicians rarely feel comfortable doing this, they usually settle for recording only the peak and trough pulse rates during and after performance of the maneuver. This cannot diagnose baroreflex-sympathoneural failure.

The finding of abnormal blood pressure responses to the Valsalva maneuver is valuable for diagnosing sympathetic neurocirculatory failure (orthostatic hypotension associated with baroreflex-sympathoneural failure) but is of no value in the differential diagnosis of autonomic failure syndromes. The same abnormal pattern occurs in Parkinson's disease with orthostatic hypotension (PD+OH), pure autonomic failure (PAF), and multiple system atrophy (MSA).

Tilt table testing

Tilt table testing is done to see if standing up (orthostasis) provokes a progressive fall in blood pressure (orthostatic hypotension), an excessive increase in heart rate (as in postural tachycardia syndrome (POTS)), a sudden fall in blood pressure (neurally mediated hypotension), a prolonged period with no electrocardiographic signal (asystole), or presyncope (near fainting).The testing is quite safe when done by experienced personnel, in a setting where emergency backup is available.

The testing itself is relatively simple. The patient lies on a stretcher-like table, security straps are attached around the upper abdomen and legs, and the patient is tilted upright at an angle.

The exact angle used varies from center to center and may be from 60° to 90°. The tilting goes on for up to about 40 minutes (this again varies from center to center).

For evaluating possible neurogenic orthostatic hypotension (nOH), 5 minutes of tilting should suffice. If there were a relatively small increase in heart rate while the blood pressure was falling, this would confirm nOH. For evaluating possible POTS or autonomically mediated syncope in a patient with chronic orthostatic intolerance, a relatively long period of tilting is used. The tilting is a form of provocative test. The doctors are hoping to reproduce the patient's problem in a controlled laboratory situation.

As soon as the test becomes positive, such as by a sudden fall in blood pressure (this has been called neurally mediated hypotension or tilt-evoked hypotension), the patient is put back down to the supine position. Sometimes fluid is given by vein. Consciousness, if lost, rapidly returns; however, symptoms such as clouded thinking, a vague sense of imbalance or disorientation, or headache can persist for hours or even days later.

There are some disadvantages to tilt table testing. One is false- positive test results. In a false-positive test, the results of the test are positive, but some healthy people can have a positive test result, so that a positive test result might not actually mean that anything really is "wrong." A positive result could lead the doctor to conclude incorrectly that the condition is merely fainting, a relatively benign situation, whereas the patient may actually have a serious medical problem. Tilt table testing might also not reproduce the patient's problem—a false-negative test result.

Another disadvantage is that most tilt table testing does not provide information about disease mechanisms. This means that, beyond verifying the patient's complaints, the testing does little to suggest pathophysiologically rational treatments that might be effective. "Augmented" tilt table testing involves measurements of physiological functions such as forearm vascular resistance and blood sampling for assays of levels of NE and EPI. Augmented testing can provide information about mechanisms; however, few centers offer this form of tilt table testing.

Sweat tests

Sweating plays an important role in the regulation of body temperature when a person is exposed to environmental heat.

The brain increases sweating by directing an increase in sympathetic cholinergic system (SCS) traffic to sweat glands in the skin. The chemical messenger, acetylcholine, is released, the acetylcholine occupies muscarinic receptors on the sweat glands, and the glands secrete sweat. This promotes evaporative heat loss.

One can examine SCS function from the sweating response to external heat—the thermoregulatory sweat test, or TST. Sweat production can be visualized by sprinkling starch with iodine or other indicator powder (e.g., alizarin red) all over the body and testing the patient in a heat chamber. When the powder is wetted because of perspiration the powder turns color. One can then photograph the body and see which parts sweated. This sort of sweat testing can be informative in detecting small fiber neuropathy, sympathetic cholinergic denervation in the feet or hands, or denervation in large areas of the trunk.

Sweating increases local humidity, and one can monitor the humidity in a chamber strapped to a limb and applied to the skin. One can also take pictures of sweat droplets or obtain a latex impression of the droplets to quantify the amount of sweating.

When the skin becomes sweaty, the ability to conduct electricity increases because of the salt and water in the sweat, and one can monitor the electrical conductivity. The galvanic skin response (GSR), or skin sympathetic test (SST), is part of polygraphic "lie detector" testing. When a person is startled or a small electric shock is delivered, increased sweating is detected by the increase in skin electrical conductance (SEC).

These sweat tests are generally safe. A disadvantage is that they mainly or only measure physiological changes as a result of release of acetylcholine from sympathetic nerves. That is, they assess only one component of the autonomic nervous system. The TST cannot distinguish sympathetic cholinergic denervation from a lesion in central neural pathways involved in thermoregulation. Carrying out the TST requires a specialized heat chamber that is not available at many centers. Commonly used drugs for urinary incontinence block acetylcholine receptors and can interfere with the results of the TST.

A common sweat test is the quantitative sudomotor axon reflex test (QSART). Because the test involves administration of a drug (acetylcholine), the QSART is described later in the section on pharmacological tests.

Pupillometry

Pupillometry involves tracking the dynamics of pupil size in response to a brief light stimulus. This is a simple, non-invasive autonomic function test.

In response to a brief light stimulus, the pupils constrict due to a rapid increase in parasympathetic nervous system (PNS) activity. After the light stimulus, the pupils slowly re-dilate.

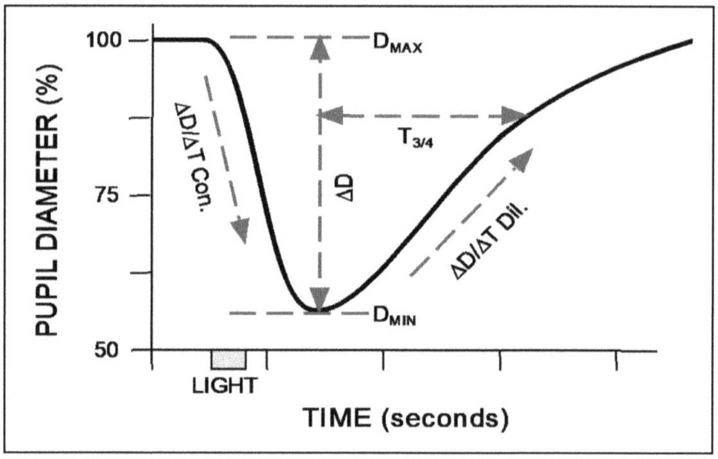

Some measurement parameters in pupillometry.

The re-dilation involves a contribution of the sympathetic noradrenergic system (SNS), since patients with Horner's syndrome (discussed below) not only have a small pupil but also have a delay in the return of pupil diameter toward baseline (prolonged T3/4 in Fig. 243). The pupillary light reflex is too rapid to involve adrenaline.

How pupillometry results relate to abnormalities of particular components of the autonomic nervous system is a matter of current research.

Horne's syndrome (also called Horner-Bernard and Bernard-Horner syndrome depending on your loyalty to Claude Bernard) involves the triad of ptosis (lid lag), miosis (constricted pupils), and anhidrosis (lack of sweating) on the affected side of the face. Horner's syndrome usually reflects loss of input from the sympathetic noradrenergic system (SNS) and sympathetic cholinergic system (SCS), so that parasympathetic nervous system (PNS) effects on the pupils are unopposed. Sympathetic nerves to the face travel from the thoracic spinal cord through ganglia before ascending in the chest and neck to the head. A tumor in the chest or neck that impinges on the sympathetic chain can manifest clinically as Horner's syndrome.

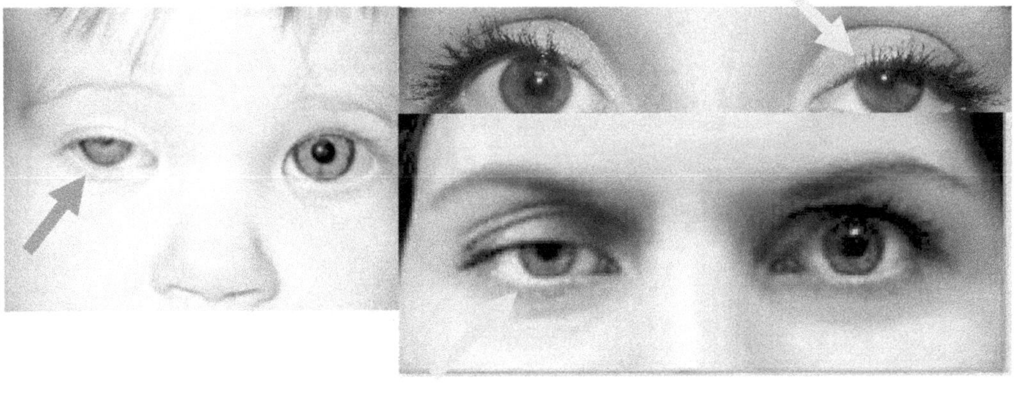

Examples of Horner's syndrome.

Ambulatory blood pressure monitoring

Ambulatory blood pressure monitoring, or ABPM, refers to automatic recording of blood pressure at pre-set time intervals during activities of daily life.

ABPM done over 24 hours can be valuable to assess whether the patient has the normal "dipping" of blood pressure that occurs during the night. Non-dipping often occurs in patients with neurogenic orthostatic hypotension, because during the day the patients have relatively low blood pressure when they are upright, and at night they have relatively high blood pressure when they are lying down (supine hypertension).

ABPM is quite useful to assess variability of blood pressure over hours of observation. Patients with arterial baroreflex failure typically have large swings of blood pressure during the day and night.

Some patients have "white coat hypertension," meaning their blood pressures are high in the doctor's office but are normal at home. ABPM can also help diagnose white coat hypertension.

Gastric emptying

Many autonomic, endocrine, and local factors regulate stomach emptying after ingestion of a meal. The term, "gastroparesis," refers to delayed gastric emptying due to poor stomach motility.

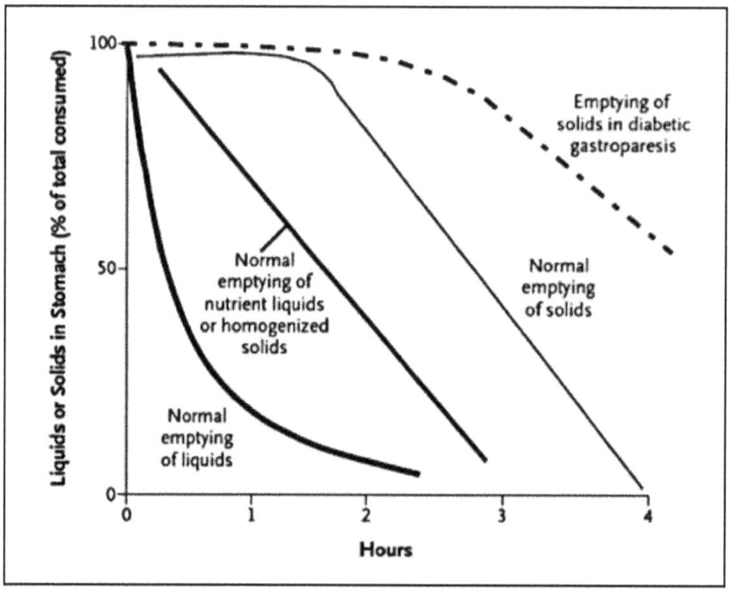

Gastric emptying times.

A decreased rate of gastric emptying can be a sign of parasympathetic nervous system (PNS) failure, sympathetic noradrenergic system (SNS) hyperactivity, increased circulating adrenaline levels, or any of a variety of endocrine or local enteric neuronal abnormalities. One clinical test of gastric emptying is based on nuclear medical scanning after swallowing a substance tagged with radioactivity.

Probably the most common disorders involving gastroparesis are diabetes mellitus, Parkinson's disease, and multiple sclerosis. Gastroparesis can also result from damage during gastric surgery to branches of the vagus nerve that supply the stomach.

The cold pressor test

In the cold pressor test, blood pressure is monitored when the patient dunks a hand into a bucket of ice-cold water and keeps the hand immersed. This rapidly increases the blood pressure by increasing activity of the sympathetic noradrenergic system (SNS). In a patient with baroreflex failure and an intact SNS, the cold pressor test would be expected to evoke an exaggerated increase in blood pressure, while in a patient with baroreflex failure and loss of sympathetic noradrenergic nerves the pressor response would be blunted.

The cold pressor test can only be done for a minute or two. The stimulus is complex and dynamic because of the rapid development of pain, numbness, and distress. Patients with dysautonomia associated with chronic burning pain in the skin (erythromelalgia) can have a remarkable ability to tolerate prolonged cold pressor testing.

Pharmacological Tests

Pharmacological tests of the autonomic nervous system (ANS) involve giving a drug and measuring its effects on physiological measures of ANS functions or on levels of a biochemical such as NE. There always is at least some risk of side effects of test drugs. In addition, test drugs can interact with medications the patient is on to treat the disease or with other conditions the patient has.

Sometimes results of pharmacological tests can be as difficult to interpret as those of physiologic tests. For instance, a pharmacological test of the role of the sympathetic noradrenergic system (SNS) in a person's high blood pressure (BP) might include measuring the effects of a drug that blocks sympathetic nerve traffic on BP, because a large fall in BP would suggest an important role of the SNS in keeping the BP high. But if blocking the sympathetic nerve traffic compensatorily activated another system that also increased BP, then the sympathetic blocking drug would not decrease the pressure, and the doctor might mistakenly think that the SNS wasn't involved with the patient's high BP.

The QSART

"QSART" stands for "Quantitative Sudomotor Axon Reflex Test." This test is a special form of sweat test to determine the ability of sympathetic nerves in the skin to release endogenous acetylcholine and increase sweat production.

In the QSART, dried air is pumped through a small plastic capsule placed on the skin. When the person sweats, the humidity in the chamber increases. This provides a measure of sweat production.

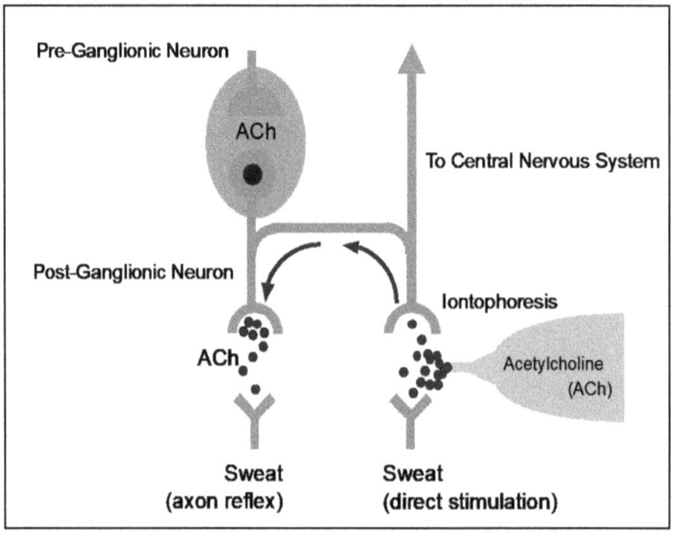

In the quantitative sudomotor axon reflex test (QSART) local humidity is measured after iontophoresis of acetylcholine at the skin's surface.

For QSART testing, acetylcholine (ACh) is applied to the skin by a special procedure called iontophoresis, in which a small amount of electricity enables the acetylcholine to penetrate the skin. The locally applied ACh evokes sweating at the site where it is given, but in addition, by way of a type of reflex called an axon reflex, sympathetic nerves under the plastic capsule release the body's own (endogenous) ACh. This results in sweat production measured by increased humidity in the capsule.

If a person had a loss of sympathetic cholinergic nerves in the region being tested, then applying ACh to the skin around the test capsule would not lead to increased sweating or increased humidity in the test capsule. If the person had a brain disease that prevented increases in sympathetic cholinergic nerve traffic during exposure to increased environmental temperature, then the person would not be able to increase the humidity in the capsule in response to an increase in the room temperature, yet the person would have a normal QSART response. This combination of findings occurs in some patients with multiple system atrophy. By this sort of combined neuropharmacological/physiological test doctors can distinguish sympathetic cholinergic system (SCS) failure due to loss of sympathetic cholinergic nerves from failure due to abnormal regulation of nerve traffic in intact nerves.

Advantages of the QSART are that it is generally safe, quick, quantitative, and easy to perform; however, the equipment is expensive. As in other tests where the dependent measure is physiological (in this case, sweat production), the results are indirect. If the patient had a decreased ability to synthesize or store ACh in sympathetic cholinergic nerve terminals, decreased numbers of ACh receptors on the sweat-secreting cells, or decreased numbers of sweat glands, the patient would have the same abnormal QSART responses as if the sympathetic cholinergic nerves were lost. QSART results may not identify problems with other components of the autonomic nervous system.

QSART testing is used also to detect a loss of autonomic nerve fibers in the feet, as occurs in small fiber neuropathies and "neuropathic" POTS.

Tyramine testing

In the tyramine (TYR) infusion test, the drug tyramine is infused intravenously (IV). TYR that is taken up into the sympathetic nerves displaces norepinephrine (NE) from the vesicles. Some of the NE reaches its receptors on vascular smooth muscle cells, and the blood pressure goes up.

If a patient had autonomic failure due to a loss of sympathetic nerves, TYR would not release NE from the nerves, because there would be no NE to displace. In such a patient TYR would not increase the blood pressure by as much as if the patient had an intact sympathetic noradrenergic system (SNS). In addition, such a patient would have relatively small increases in levels of NE and related compounds, such as DHPG, in the plasma.

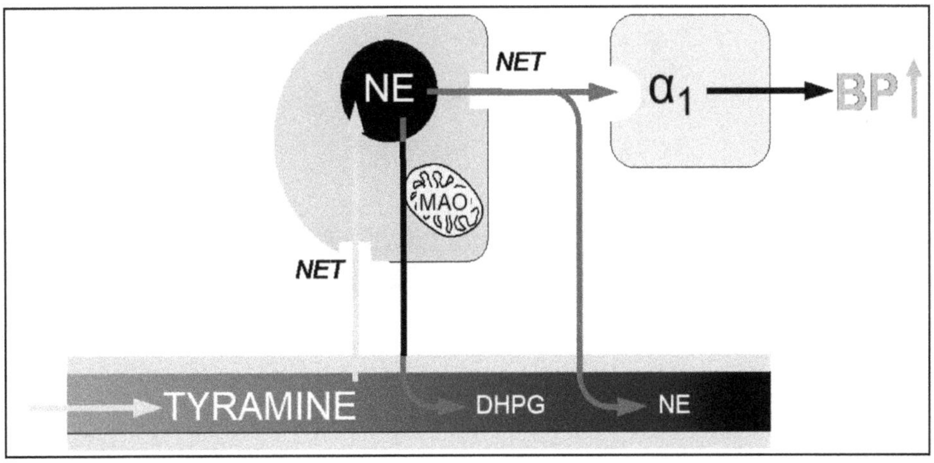

Effects of infused tyramine on blood pressure and plasma levels of NE and DHPG.

Clonidine suppression Test

Clonidine (brand name Catapres™) is an imidazoline that stimulates alpha-2 adrenoceptors in the brain, in blood vessel walls, and on sympathetic nerves. Clonidine decreases blood pressure (BP) by two mechanisms—inhibiting sympathetic noradrenergic system (SNS) outflows and inhibiting norepinephrine (NE) release for a given amount of SNS traffic. Although stimulation of alpha-2 adrenoceptors on vascular smooth muscle cells would be expected to increase BP, but this effect usually is overwhelmed by the other effects, and except in rare situations clonidine drops the BP.

The clonidine suppression test is based on effects of the drug on BP and on plasma levels of NE. If a patient had excessive activity of the sympathetic noradrenergic system (SNS), then clonidine would produce large decreases in BP and plasma NE levels. Clonidine suppression testing therefore can identify long-term high BP associated with increased release of NE from sympathetic nerve terminals—hypernoradrenergic hypertension.

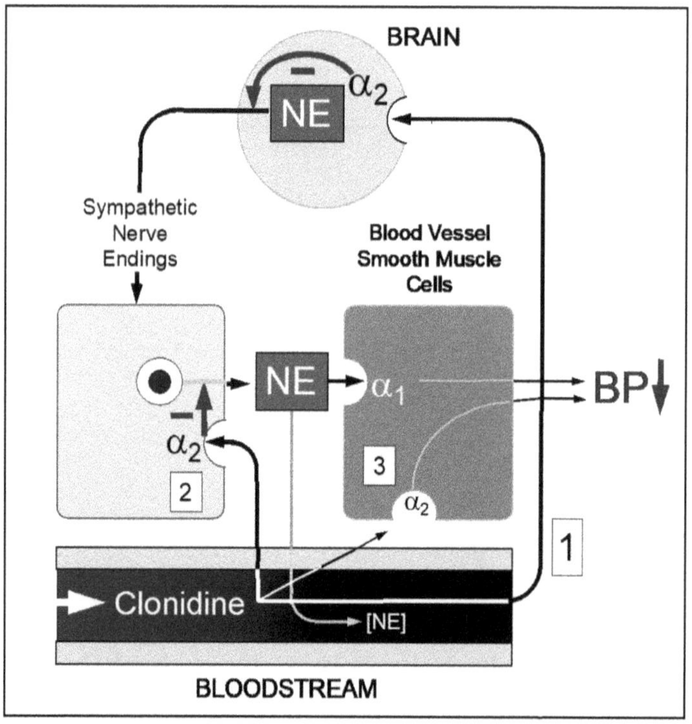

Processes involved with the clonidine suppression test. The drug decreases blood pressure (BP) by (1) decreasing sympathetic noradrenergic outflow and (2) inhibiting norepinephrine release. Ordinarily these inhibitory effects are greater than the direct stimulatory effect (3) at alpha-2 adrenoceptors on vascular smooth muscle cells.

Clonidine suppression testing is used mainly to evaluate possible pheochromocytoma, a tumor that produces catecholamines. In pheochromocytoma the plasma NE levels fail to decrease after clonidine administration, due to continuous, unregulated NE secretion by the tumor.

Neurochemical Tests

Neurochemical tests involve measuring levels of body chemicals, such as the catecholamines norepinephrine (NE) and epinephrine (EPI), either under resting conditions, in response to physiological manipulations such as exercise and head-up tilt, or in response to a pharmacological manipulation. Neurochemical tests themselves are safe, but the type of body fluid sampling, such as arterial blood sampling or cerebrospinal fluid sampling after a lumbar puncture, can involve some risk. The results can be affected importantly by diet, posture, drugs or dietary supplements the patient is taking, and the environmental conditions at the time of sampling. Moreover, relatively few centers have a clinical neurochemistry laboratory to carry out the relevant assays.

There is no neurochemical test of parasympathetic nervous system (PNS) activity. This is because acetylcholine (ACh), the chemical messenger of the PNS, is broken down by an enzyme almost as soon as ACh enters body fluids such as the plasma. There are indirect measures, such as pancreatic polypeptide levels.

Some blood tests involve measuring levels not of neurochemicals but of factors in the circulation that affect the functioning of one or more components of the autonomic nervous system. For instance, there are uncommon forms of dysautonomia in which there are high titers of antibodies to the nicotinic cholinergic receptor that is required for relaying signals in the autonomic ganglia.

Neurochemical tests of autonomic nervous system functions are mainly done to examine activities of the sympathetic noradrenergic system (SNS) and the sympathetic adrenergic system (SAS). This is because the main chemical messengers of these systems, NE and EPI, can be measured in the plasma.

The cat comes back

In the diagnostic evaluation of patients with known or suspected dysautonomias, measurement of plasma catechols are rarely diagnostic but often are informative. Measurements of the intra-neuronal metabolites with the parent compounds can greatly enhance the information compared to measuring the catecholamines alone.

Human plasma normally contains at least 7 catechols. Three are the catecholamines NE, EPI, and dopamine. Another is 3,4-dihydroxyphenylalanine (DOPA), which is the precursor of the catecholamines and the immediate product of the rate-limiting enzyme in catecholamine biosynthesis, tyrosine hydroxylase (TH). DOPA is converted to dopamine by the enzymatic action of L-aromatic-amino-acid decarboxylase (LAAAD). 3,4-Dihydroxyphenylglycol (DHPG) is the main intra- neuronal metabolite of norepinephrine, and 3,4- dihydroxyphenylacetic acid (DOPAC) is the main intra-neuronal metabolite of DA. Both are formed from the enzymatic action of monoamine oxidase (MAO) on cytoplasmic catecholamines. Another endogenous catechol typically found in human plasma is 5-S-cysteinylDOPA (Cys-DOPA). Cys-DOPA is formed from covalent bonding of DOPA with cysteine (or with glutathione, followed by enzymatic conversion of glutathione to cysteine). Plasma Cys-DOPA is high in patients with renal failure.

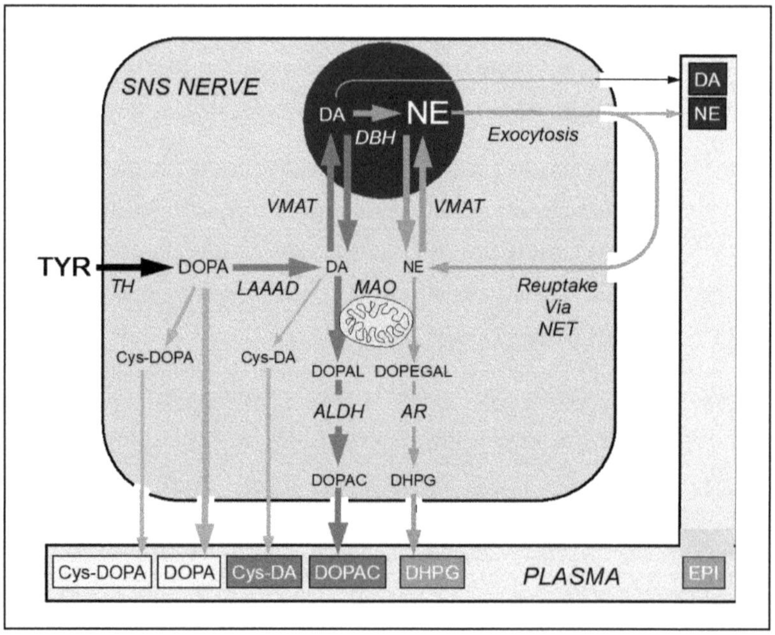

Plasma levels of catechols are related to particular processes in sympathetic noradrenergic nerves.

Plasma norepinephrine (NE)

Since norepinephrine (NE) is the main chemical messenger of the sympathetic noradrenergic system (SNS), the plasma NE level has often been used as an index of SNS "activity" in the body as a whole. In people who are resting lying down, plasma NE levels normally range from about 100 to about 500 pg/mL.

Condition	Catechol Pattern
DBH deficiency	Low NE, DHPG
	High DA, DOPAC
Menkes disease	High DOPA/DHPG
	High DA/NE
LAAAD deficiency	High DOPA/DOPAC
	High DOPA/DA
HSAN III (FD)	High DOPA/DHPG

Measuring plasma catechols is diagnostic in some rare conditions.

Condition	Catechol Pattern
Diabetic autonomic neuropathy	Low DHPG/NE
POTS	High upright NE
Neurally mediated hypotension	High EPI/NE during tilt
PD+OH	Blunted orthostatic %ΔNE
Diabetic autonomic neuropathy	Low DHPG/NE
DLB	Blunted orthostatic %ΔNE
Takotsubo cardiopathy	High EPI
PAF	Low NE, DHPG, blunted ortho. %ΔNE
Pseudopheo	High EPI after glucagon
Famil. amyloid. polyneuropathy	Low NE, blunted ortho. %ΔNE
HSAN IV	Low NE
Pheo	High NE, blunted clonidine suppression

Measuring plasma catechols often is informative, such as in the above conditions.

The relationship between the rate of sympathetic nerve traffic and the concentration of norepinephrine in the plasma is complex and indirect and is influenced by many factors. The blood sample should be obtained under carefully controlled or monitored conditions, and the plasma NE level should be interpreted by an expert.

Plasma epinephrine (EPI)

Compared to the plasma NE level, which is complexly and indirectly related to overall sympathetic noradrenergic system (SNS) activity in the body as a whole, the plasma EPI (adrenaline) level is a fairly direct indicator of activity of the sympathetic adrenergic system (SAS).

Nevertheless, some factors can complicate interpreting plasma EPI levels. When the blood flow in the arm or hand is slow, there is greater extraction of the arterial EPI during its passage through the tissues. In the setting of high forearm vascular resistance, the EPI level in the antecubital venous plasma underestimates the level in the arterial plasma.

A large number of common and difficult to control life experiences influence activity of the SAS. These include drugs, alterations in blood glucose levels (such as after a meal), body temperature, posture, and especially emotional distress.

An additional problem is technical. Because EPI is a very powerful hormone, the plasma level normally is very low–so low that it is often below the limit of detection of commercially available laboratory assays. In a healthy person lying down, plasma EPI levels can be as low as a few picograms (a millionth of a millionth of a gram) per milliliter.

Finally, other chemicals besides EPI can interfere with the measurement. This can especially be a problem in people who drink a lot of coffee, even if it is decaffeinated, because of chemicals in the plasma that can mimic EPI in the assay procedure.

Plasma 3,4-dihydroxyphenylglycol (DHPG)

DHPG is the main neuronal metabolite of NE. Combined measurements of plasma DHPG and NE can offer insights about processes in sympathetic noradrenergic nerves that measurement of NE alone cannot provide.

For instance, in a patients with postural tachycardia syndrome, high plasma NE levels have been used to diagnose "hyperadrenergic" POTS. If high plasma NE reflected diffusely increased sympathetic noradrenergic system (SNS) outflows, then plasma DHPG would be high as well; however, if high plasma NE reflected decreased neuronal reuptake of NE by the cell membrane NE transporter, then plasma NE would be high, but plasma DHPG would not.

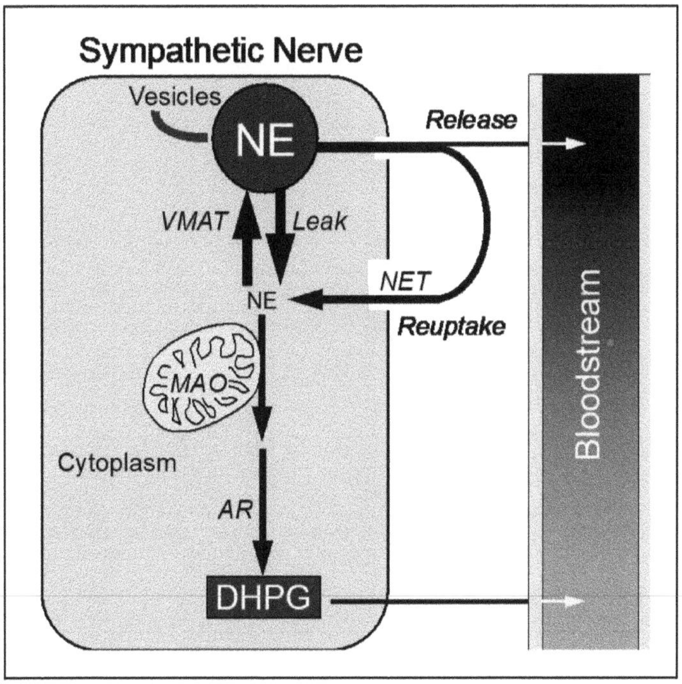

Combined measurements of NE and DHPG can separate increased sympathetic outflow from decreased neuronal reuptake as determinants of high plasma NE.

Neuroimaging Tests

Neuroimaging tests involve visualizing the autonomic nerve supply in body organs.

Cardiac sympathetic neuroimaging

Cardiac sympathetic noradrenergic neuroimaging is done commonly in Japan and Europe but rarely in the United States, even though this type of testing can produce informative images of the sympathetic innervation of the heart. Usually, sympathetic neuroimaging provides only anatomic information about whether sympathetic nerves are present in the heart. It is more difficult to determine whether the nerves that are present are functioning normally or not.

The most commonly used neuroimaging technology for visualizing cardiac sympathetic innervation is ^{123}I-metaiodobenzylguanidine (^{123}I-MIBG) single photon emission tomography (SPECT).

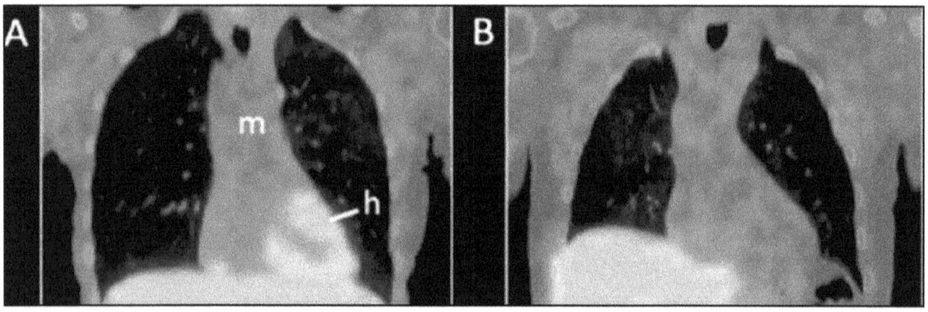

^{123}I-MIBG SPECT scans of a control subject and a patient with cardiac noradrenergic deficiency. The heart/mediastinum (h/m) ratio of radioactivity is used as a quantitative measure of sympathetic innervation.

^{18}F-Dopamine positron emission tomography (PET) is superior to ^{123}I-MIBG SPECT in a few ways but is only available at the NIH Clinical Center.

Perhaps by learning about this technology especially for distinguishing Lewy body from non-Lewy body forms of autonomic failure you might convince decision-makers at academic centers to do ^{18}F-dopamine PET!

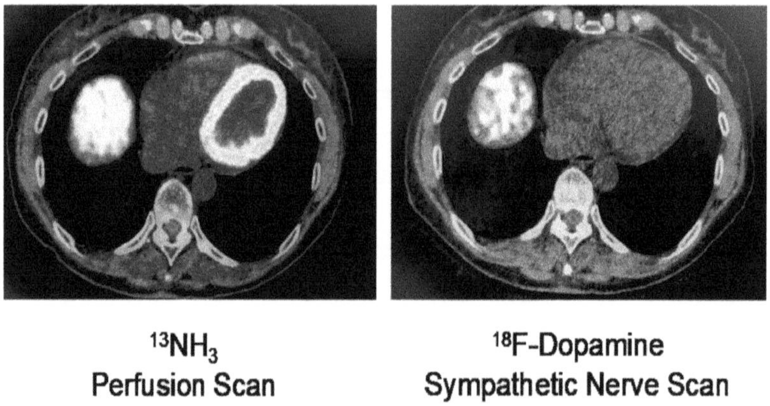

^{18}F-Dopamine positron emission tomography (PET) is a powerful way to visualize sympathetic noradrenergic innervation of the heart. The ^{13}N-ammonia perfusion scan of the same patient shows where the heart is.

Central catecholaminergic neuroimaging

Central nervous system neuroimaging by "DAT" scans or ^{18}F-DOPA PET can identify brain diseases associated with dysautonomias, such as Parkinson's disease with neurogenic orthostatic hypotension. DAT stands for the cell membrane dopamine transporter (DAT). ^{18}F-DOPA is a neutral amino acid and enters all cells, whether or not they express the DAT. Within cells that express L-aromatic-amino-acid decarboxylase (LAAAD), ^{18}F-DOPA is converted to ^{18}F-dopamine, and in nerve terminals that express the vesicular monoamine transporter (VMAT), the ^{18}F-dopamine is taken up into the vesicles.

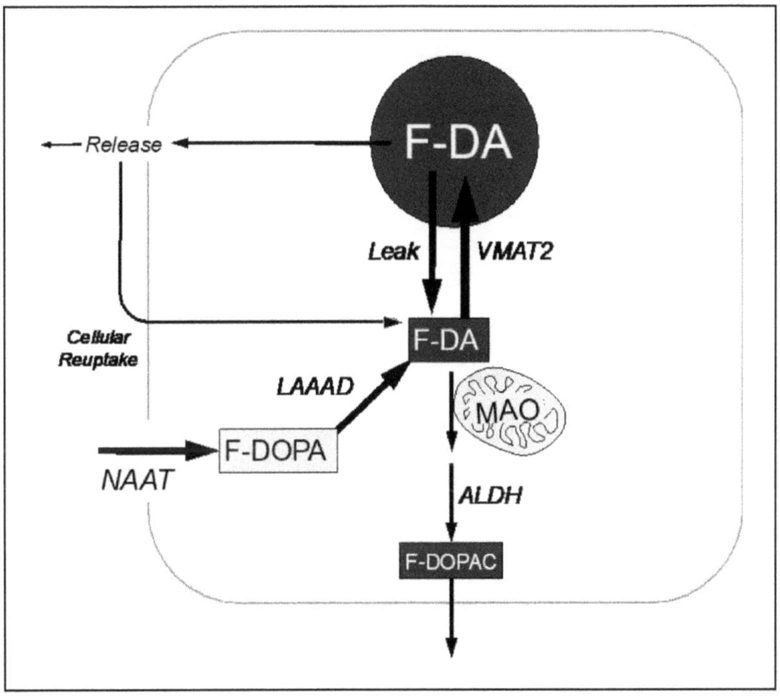

The basis for ^{18}F-DOPA PET scanning is uptake via the neutral amino acid transporter (NAAT), enzymatic decarboxylation by LAAAD to form ^{18}F-dopamine (^{18}F-DA), and uptake of the ^{18}F-dopamine into storage vesicles.

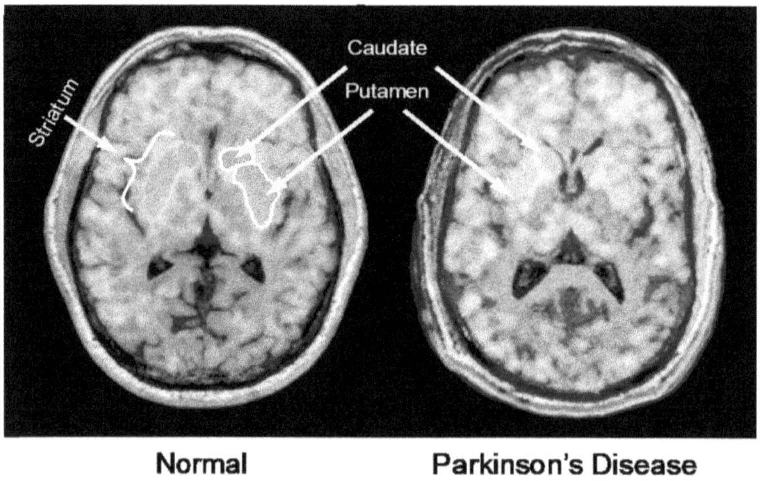

^{18}F-DOPA PET can identify loss of striatal dopaminergic terminals such as in Parkinson's disease.

Other Tests

Skin biopsies

The dermis of the skin contains three constituents that receive post-ganglionic sympathetic innervation—sweat glands, arrector pili (pilomotor) muscles, and blood vessels. There have been major recent advances in visualizing the nerves supplying these structures and using the images as biomarkers of specific forms of dysautonomia.

The sweat glands in the skin receive sympathetic cholinergic nerve fibers. These post-ganglionic, non-myelinated, slow- conducting fibers release acetylcholine. The acetylcholine binds to muscarinic receptors, evoking sweat secretion. In skin biopsy samples, one can identify the sympathetic cholinergic fibers by their contents of vaso-active intestinal peptide (VIP) or choline acetyltransferase (ChAT).

The hair follicles have small muscles attached to them called pilomotor or arrector pili muscles. The pilomotor muscles are responsible for the hair standing up, or piloerection, when you are exposed to cold or when you are distressed. The muscles receive sympathetic noradrenergic nerve fibers relatively specifically. The nerves release norepinephrine, which binds to alpha-adrenoceptors on the arrector pili muscles, and the hair stands up.

In skin biopsy samples, one can identify sympathetic noradrenergic fibers by their contents of dopamine-beta- hydroxylase (DBH) or tyrosine hydroxylase (TH).

Since the arrector pili muscles and the walls of blood vessels receive purely sympathetic noradrenergic innervation, PGP 9.5 staining can identify sympathetic noradrenergic nerves in these structures, even though PGP 9.5

reacts with all forms of small nerve fibers, not just post-ganglionic autonomic fibers. Examining nerves in skin biopsy specimens can be considered to be a form of microscopic autonomic neuroimaging. Examination of nerve fibers in the epidermis provides a way to identify small fiber neuropathy. This usually is done by staining for the non-specific axonal marker, protein gene product 9.5, or PGP 9.5. PGP 9.5 staining cannot easily distinguish sensory from autonomic fibers.

Three types of skin constituents in the dermis receive autonomic post-ganglionic innervation—sweat glands, blood vessels, and arrector pili (pilomotor) muscles.

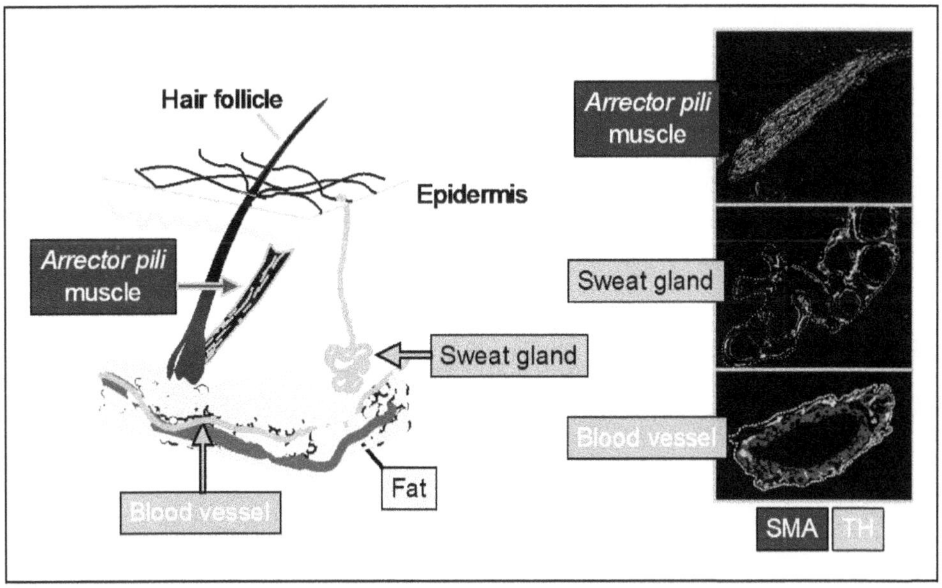

Three sympathetic noradrenergically innervated structures—arrector pili (pilomotor) muscles, sweat glands, and blood vessels.

Sweat glands receive sympathetic cholinergic fibers, which can be identified specifically by staining for immunoreactive vasoactive intestinal peptide (VIP) or choline acetyltransferase (ChAT). Sweat glands also have sympathetic noradrenergic fibers, which identified by specifically staining for immunoreactive dopamine-beta-hydroxylase (DBH) or tyrosine hydroxylase (TH). Since blood vessels and arrector pili muscles receive sympathetic noradrenergic innervation exclusively, PGP 9.5 staining of these structures can be used to assess the status of local sympathetic noradrenergic innervation.

Genetic tests

The area of genetic testing in autonomic medicine is rapidly expanding. In autosomal dominantly transmitted diseases, even one copy of a mutated gene is sufficient to produce the disease. One-half the family members will inherit the mutation and have the disease (assuming perfect "penetrance"). In autosomal recessive diseases, both parents are carriers. Since each parent donates one chromosome, the chances are 25% that their offspring will have the disease. An X-linked recessive disease involves a mutation on the X chromosome. The disease is expressed in males but not in females, because in females the other X chromosome does not carry the mutation. The mothers of boys with an X-linked recessive inherited disease are carriers. If a known carrier is pregnant with a boy, the chances are 50% that he will have the disease.

In general, the more common the genetic alteration in the population, the lower the risk associated with that alteration.

Genetic tests involve several ethical issues. For instance, it is difficult to ensure confidentiality of the data when patient pedigrees are published or available from data repositories. An individual may not wish to be informed of the test result if there is no way to prevent the disease. Researchers may be reluctant to provide results of genetic tests if the laboratory is not certified to do diagnostic testing.

The following text highlights some dysautonomias or catecholamine-related disorders involving genetic mutations:

- The most well-known inherited dysautonomia is familial dysautonomia (FD), or Riley-Day syndrome. FD runs in families of Ashkenazi extraction. The cause is a mutation of the gene, IKBKAP.
- A rare cause of orthostatic hypotension is deficiency of the enzyme, dopamine-beta-hydroxylase (DBH), which is required to produce NE.
- Postural tachycardia syndrome (POTS) can result from mutation of the gene that encodes the cell membrane norepinephrine transporter (NET). Although POTS is common, POTS from this genetic cause is very rare.

can be

- Menkes disease is a rare disease of copper metabolism.
- Because DBH is a copper enzyme, Menkes disease involves decreased NE production.
- The Menkes disease is on the X chromosome. This means that Menkes disease is transmitted as an X-linked recessive trait.
- The first identified genetic cause of PD was mutation of the gene encoding the protein, alpha-synuclein (⊠S), in 1997. The discovery was in a Greek-Italian-American kindred in which PD was transmitted as an autosomal dominant trait.

People who carry the mutation that produces Gaucher disease are at increased risk of developing PD.

Antibody tests

In autonomic autoimmunity proteins expressed in the autonomic nervous system are targeted by antibodies or immune cells.

Probably the most well characterized form of autoimmune attack is autoimmune autonomic neuropathy from a circulating antibodies targeting the neuronal nicotinic receptor. Since ganglionic neurotransmission depends on this receptor, autoimmune autonomic neuropathy manifests with decreased functions of post-ganglionic nerves. In autoimmune autonomic ganglionopathy (AAG), the attack is sufficiently severe and generalized to cause all components of the autonomic nervous system to fail clinically—a "pandysautonomia."

Cancer cells can produce antibodies to proteins expressed by autonomic nerves ("paraneoplastic syndrome"). Anti-Hu ntibodies (also known as Type 1 anti-neuronal nuclear antibody, ANNA-1) are especially common in small cell lung cancers.

A variety of infectious diseases can result in autonomic neuropathies, such as mononucleosis, herpes simplex, and Coxsackie B.

Lambert-Eaton myasthenic syndrome is an autoimmune disorder of neuromuscular transmission characterized by antibodies directed against presynaptic, voltage-gated calcium channels, impairing acetylcholine release. This syndrome is most commonly associated with symptoms and signs of parasympathetic nervous system failure. Several diseases can include autonomic neuropathy that may have an autoimmune mechanism, such as diabetes, Guillain- Barré syndrome, Sjogren's syndrome, lupus, and amyloidosis. In general, there is no specific test to identify the specific offending antibody. These are discussed later in this book. It should be noted that the presence of an antibody, such as to the neuronal nicotinic receptor, does not mean that the antibody is pathogenic and causes or contributes to dysautonomia. It can be very difficult to make this determination with confidence.

One way to assess this possibility is by plasma exchange. In this procedure, the patient's blood is drawn into a machine that separates the cells from the plasma, removes the plasma, and infuses the patient's cells back into the patient, along with saline, albumin, and electrolytes. Plasma exchange temporarily decreases circulating levels of all antibodies. Rapid improvement in the patient's symptoms and signs would indicate that one or more antibodies are pathogenic, but it would not identify the specific antibody.

THE DYSAUTONOMIAS UNIVERSE

"Dysautonomia" refers to a condition in which altered functions of one or more components of the autonomic nervous system (ANS) adversely affect health.

Probably the most common type of dysautonomia involves compensatory, otherwise normal ANS responses that worsen an independent disease process, rather than involving an abnormality of the ANS itself. Otherwise normal changes in activities of the ANS can be harmful or even lethal in the setting of an independent disease state. A classic example is sudden death in an old man shoveling snow.

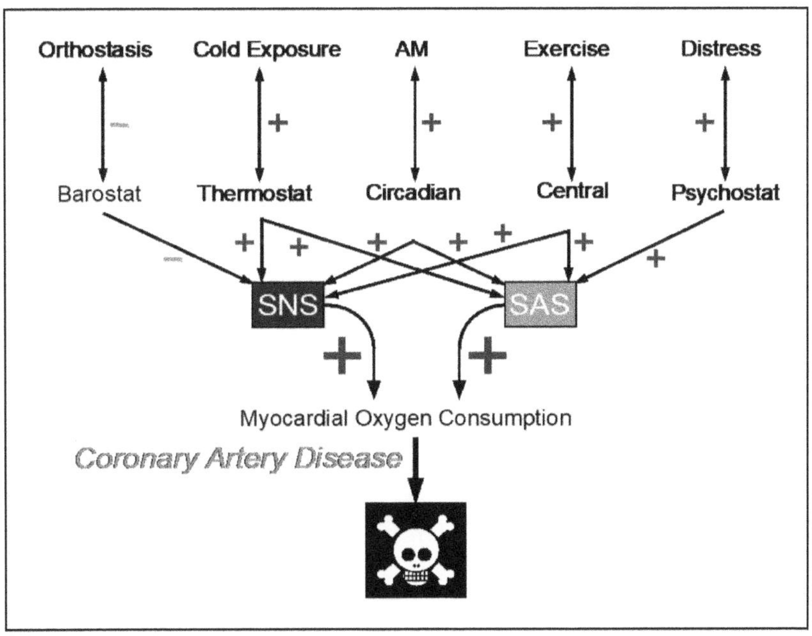

In the setting of an independent pathophysiologic state, SNS and SAS activation can be lethal.

The dysautonomias encountered in autonomic medicine usually arise from abnormal functioning within the ANS itself. This is the form of dysautonomia emphasized for the rest of this book.

Rather than being one condition there are numerous distinctive entities in an ever-expanding "dysautonomias universe." One way of conceptualizing the dysautonomias universe is to divide them into constellations by age—pediatric, adult, and geriatric.

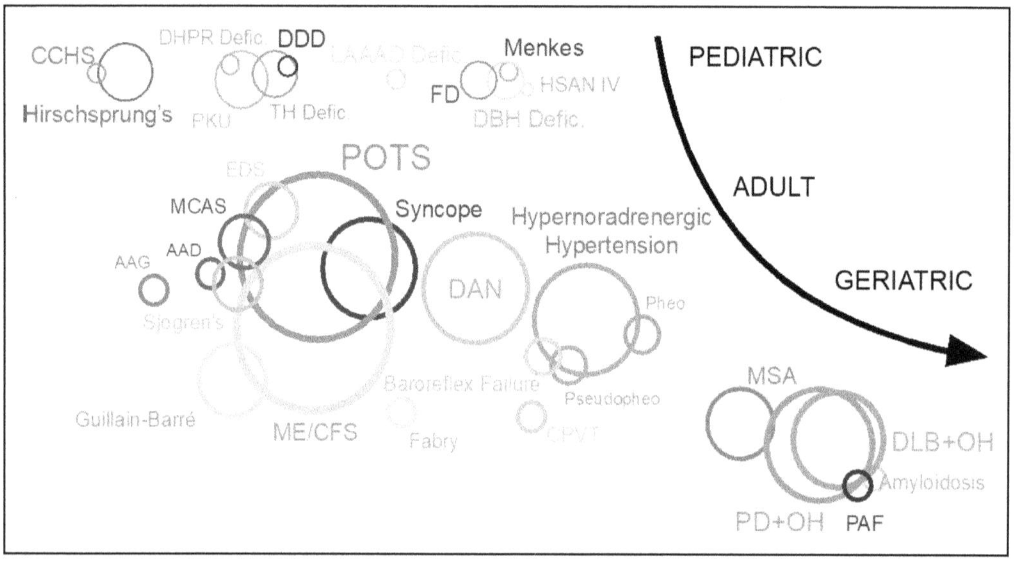

The Dysautonomias Universe. There are numerous forms of dysautonomia, which can be roughly divided by patient age group.

It is impossible in this book for students to cover all these conditions. The emphasis is on dysautonomias for which patients are referred frequently to autonomic referral centers, are important historically, or illustrate scientific principles. Dysautonomias involving abnormal cardiovascular functions have dominated research and clinical practice.

Dysautonomias in Different Age Groups

This section provides an overview of dysautonomias in different age groups.

Pediatric

Dysautonomias in infants and young children often reflect problems in ANS development. Frequently, but by no means always, the cause is a genetic abnormality such as a mutation—a "typo" in the genetic encyclopedia. A mutation found in people of Ashkenazic extraction causes familial dysautonomia (FD). Another mutation produces dysautonomias in children because of a type of phenylketonuria (PKU). Another causes "kinky hair disease" (Menkes disease). In Hirschsprung's disease, there is a lack of development of nerve cells of the enteric nervous system (ENS) in the colon, usually without an identified mutation.

Adolescent or Adult Dysautonomias

In adolescents or adults, dysautonomias frequently involve inappropriate regulation of an intact ANS. In autonomic referral centers this type of dysautonomia is especially common. Examples are autonomically mediated syncope (also called vaso-vagal syncope or neurocardiogenic syncope), in which the person suffers from frequent episodes of fainting or near fainting; and postural tachycardia syndrome (POTS), in which the person cannot tolerate being upright up for long periods and has a rapid pulse rate during standing.

Practicing internists may see patients with hypernoradrenergic hypertension, in which overactivity of the SNS causes a form of high blood pressure. Endocrinologists may see patients with pseudopheochromocytoma, which clinically resembles a rare tumor that releases catecholamines.

Dysautonomias in adults often are associated with—and may be secondary to—another disease process or a drug. Common secondary causes include medications, diabetes (diabetic autonomic neuropathy, or DAN), chemotherapy for cancer, baroreflex failure as a late sequela of irradiation of the neck, and alcoholism.

Altered activities of components of the ANS can be an attempt to compensate for dehydration, low blood volume, or excessive shifts in blood volume during orthostasis. A viral infection may impact the ANS, or autonomic nerves may be subject to autoimmune attack, as in autoimmune autonomic ganglionopathy (AAG).

There is increasing recognition of autoimmune contributions to the functional autonomic changes that occur in adolescent/adult dysautonomias. Besides AAG there are Guillain-Barré syndrome, Sjogren's syndrome, myalgic encephalitis/chronic fatigue syndrome (ME/CFS), mast cell activation syndrome (MCAS), Ehlers-Danlos syndrome (EDS), and autoimmunity-associated autonomic failure with sympathetic denervation (AAD). This currently is an area of active research.

Rarely, dysautonomias in adults can reflect genetic mutations. There is a rare form of POTS that is associated with a mutation that decreases the ability to inactivate NE, the chemical messenger of the SNS. Sympathetic neurocirculatory failure can also result from a mutation of the gene that encodes dopamine-beta-hydroxylase (DBH), which is required to synthesize NE.

Geriatric dysautonomias

In the elderly, dysautonomias typically reflect neurodegeneration. The degeneration may take the form of lesions in the central nervous system, as in multiple system atrophy (MSA), loss or dysfunction of sympathetic post-ganglionic nerves, as in pure autonomic failure (PAF), or both, as in Parkinson's disease with orthostatic hypotension (PD+OH).

Posssible Causes

The following diagrams provide examples of some of the causes of under- or over-activity of components of the ANS. It is important to recognize that for all these alterations the most common cause is drugs.

> In patients referred for dysautonomia, the first thing to do is get a complete record of all their drugs and dietary supplements. That may be the key to helping the patient.

Sympathetic noradrenergic system (SNS) hypofunction

Several drugs inhibit functions of the sympathetic noradrenergic system (SNS). These include adrenoceptor blockers, tricyclic antidepressants, clonidine, and prednisone.

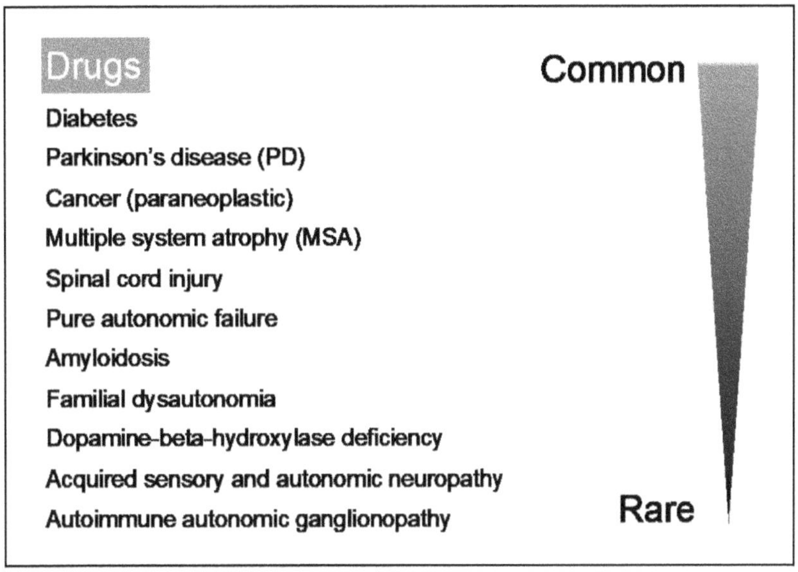

Some causes of sympathetic noradrenergic system (SNS) hypofunction.

Among diseases, diabetes probably is the most common cause of SNS underactivity, but this depends importantly on the patient age group. SNS failure may occur in the setting of a cancer or as a side effect of chemotherapy. Primary causes of SNS failure such as familial dysautonomia (FD) and autoimmune autonomic ganglionopathy (AAG) are rare.

Sympathetic noradrenergic system (SNS) hyperactivity

Excessive SNS outflow to the heart is thought to be a common theme in postural tachycardia syndrome (POTS). In hypernoradrenergic hypertension high plasma NE levels are associated with an augmented fall in blood pressure in response to alpha-2 adrenoceptor agonism by clonidine or to ganglion blockade. A key pathophysiological aspect of congestive heart failure is increased cardiac SNS outflow despite depletion of NE stores. Elevated SNS outflow is compensatory in dehydration and hypovolemia.

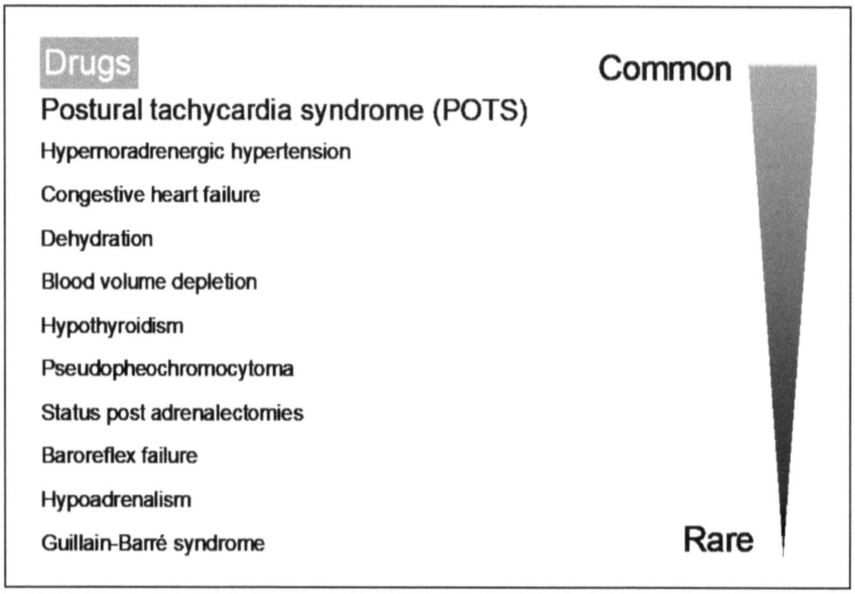

Some causes of sympathetic noradrenergic system (SNS) hyperactivity.

Parasympathetic nervous System (PNS) hypofunction

The parasympathetic nervous system (PNS) is underactive in some common conditions, including heart failure, diabetes, and Parkinson's disease.

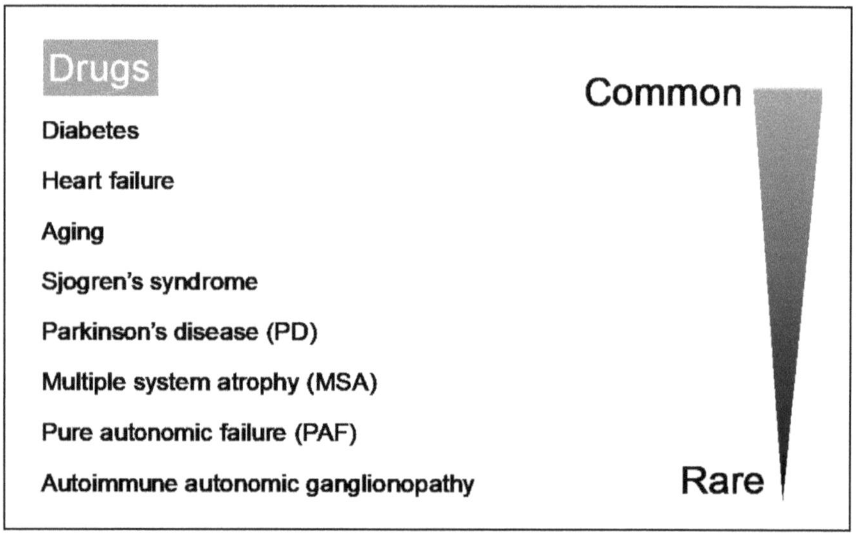

Some causes of parasympathetic nervous system (SNS) hypofunction.

PNS underactivity in these conditions probably reflects decreased neuronal outflow from the brainstem rather than loss of parasympathetic nerves. These conditions can also feature SNS underactivity (diabetes is an example) or SNS overactivity (heart failure is an example). PNS functions tend to decrease with normal aging.

Parasympathetic nervous system (PNS) hyperactivity

Increased PNS activity—especially increased vagal outflow—commonly accompanies fainting reactions ("vaso-vagal" syncope). Startle reactions entail pupillary constriction, probably mediated by increased PNS outflow. Trained athletes have relatively low heart rates.

Sympathetic adrenergic system (SAS) hyperactivity

All sensed generalized threats to organismic integrity are associated with SAS activation. Increased plasma EPI is probably the most sensitive objective biomarker of distress.

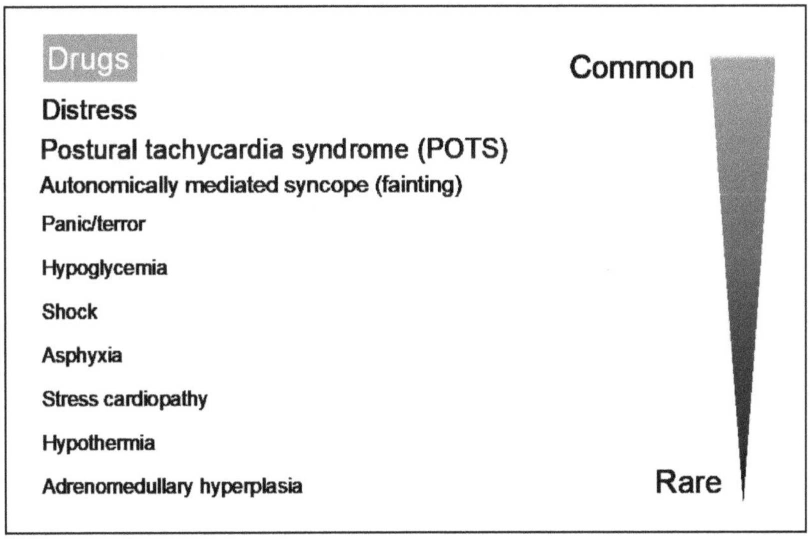

Some causes of sympathetic adrenergic system (SAS) hyperactivity.

Orthostatic Hypotension

Orthostatic hypotension (OH), a fall in blood pressure (BP) when a person stands up, is such a common sign across age groups that OH merits separate consideration. Normally when you stand up you don't notice much that is different.

Nevertheless, several automatic, largely unconscious reflexive changes are required for maintaining delivery of blood to the brain in response to this seemingly simple act. When the reflexes fail, you can't tolerate standing still while upright.

By consensus, experts define OH in terms of a fall in the systolic BP by at least 20 mmHg or a fall in diastolic BP by at least 10 mmHg between lying down and upright posture for at least 3 minutes. Doctors sometimes use different definitions, but the 20 mmHg fall in systolic BP seems to be a common theme in research reports. If the BP while lying down is very high, then more than a 20 mmHg fall in systolic pressure may be required for the doctor to diagnose OH. OH refers to a persistent, consistent problem, not to episodes. If the systolic BP persistently and consistently falls by more than 20 millimeters of mercury (mmHg) between lying on the back (supine) and standing up, this is OH. Episodic, sudden falls in BP such as from frequent fainting reactions is not OH.

> Orthostatic hypotension (OH) is defined by a fall in systolic BP by 20 mmHg or a fall in diastolic BP by10 mmHg between lying down and standing up.

OH is an important sign of failure of the sympathetic noradrenergic system (SNS). Many factors besides SNS failure can cause OH. OH can result from conditions that cause depletion of blood volume, such as heavy menstrual periods or gastrointestinal hemorrhage from a bleeding ulcer. Any of several drugs can do this, including tricyclic anti-depressants, monoamine oxidase inhibitors, and ganglion blockers.

Doctors may have different opinions about the amount of OH that is clinically significant. Normally the systolic BP falls slightly during standing up, because the heart is ejecting less blood. Normally the diastolic BP does not fall at all, because of the constriction of blood vessels in the body as a whole by way of the baroreflex and activation of the SNS.

Some people have a fall in BP accompanied by lightheadedness as soon as they get up, but then the BP comes up to normal. Most experts do not consider this immediate fall in BP to be OH, because the fall in BP is not progressive or sustained.

In neurogenic OH (nOH) the orthostatic fall in blood pressure (BP) results at least partly from an inability to increase reflexively delivery of norepinephrine (NE) to adrenoreceptors in response to a decrease in venous return to the heart. Often (but not always) nOH is accompanied by a failure to increase heart rate reflexively as the BP falls. Researchers have proposed that the extent of increase in heart rate for the decrease in systolic BP (ΔHR/ΔBPs) during orthostasis can identify nOH. Although this is a sensitive test, it is not specific. For instance, an inability to synthesize NE due to dopamine-beta-hydroxylase deficiency manifests clinically with nOH, yet ΔHR/ΔBPs is normal.

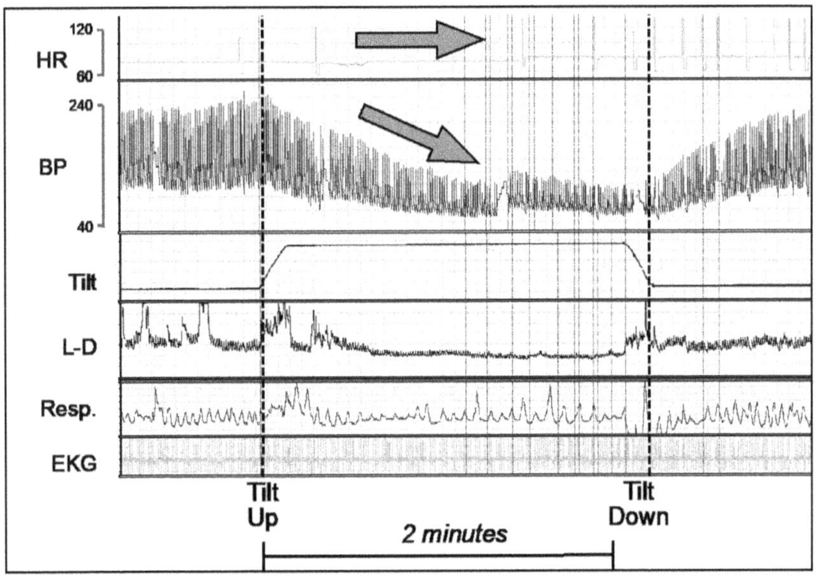

An example of neurogenic orthostatic hypotension (nOH). During head-up tilt table testing there is a progressive decrease in systolic blood pressure (BPs) that is not accompanied by an appropriate increase in heart rate (HR). A low ΔHR/ΔBPs ratio is a sensitive but not specific way to identify nOH.

Chronic Orthostatic Intolerance

There are several dysautonomias in which the patients cannot tolerate prolonged standing, even though they do not have persistent, consistent OH. These disorders come under the heading of chronic orthostatic intolerance (COI). COI can goes on for months or years.

> Patients with chronic orthostatic intolerance (COI) have a persistent inability to tolerate prolonged standing.

COI is a symptom, a complaint about something abnormal a person notices that provides subjective evidence of a disease. COI is not a sign, because it isn't something an observer can measure objectively. And it isn't a disease, although there are many diseases that produce COI.

Neither COI nor OH is a diagnosis, meaning a decision about the cause of a specific case of disease.

It is thought that about 60% of patients with chronic fatigue syndrome have COI, with postural tachycardia syndrome (POTS), autonomically mediated syncope (fainting), or both. Much less commonly, COI can be a manifestation of arterial baroreflex failure.

The fact that there are many possible causes of COI poses a challenge to doctors trying to come up with a diagnosis to explain COI in a particular patient. A starting point in identifying a cause of COI is to determine whether the patient has failure of the sympathetic noradrenergic system (SNS) to regulate the heart and blood vessels correctly. In dysautonomias that produce chronic SNS failure, the patient always has a fall in blood pressure (BP) during standing OH. In other forms of COI, the person does not have hjn **UNUU`N**sympathetic neurocirculatory failure, and the BP does not fall consistently when the person stands up (although the person can have delayed OH after many minutes of standing). Instead, the person feels dizzy or lightheaded during standing, even though the BP is maintained.

> Orthostatic hypotension (OH) may or may not produce chronic orthostatic intolerance (COI). COI usually occurs without OH.

In the evaluation of a patient with COI in which the patient does not have persistent, consistent OH, doctors often prescribe a tilt table test. Head-up tilt table testing can evoke an acute, symptomatic fall in BP. This is called neurally mediated hypotension (NMH). An alternative designation is tilt-evoked sudden hypotension (TESH), which doesn't presume a pathophysiologic mechanism.

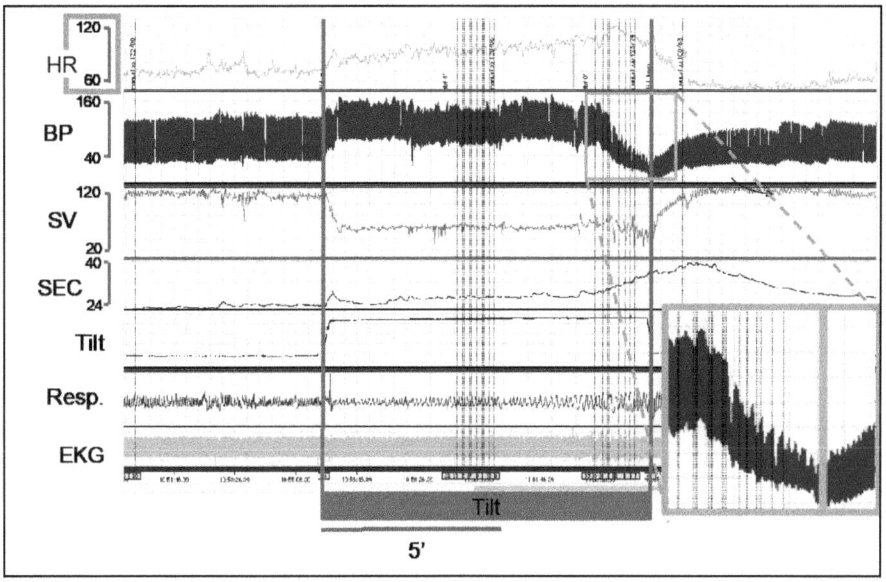

An example of excessive orthostatic tachycardia and tilt-evoked sudden hypotension in a patient with POTS.

It is usually relatively easy to distinguish OH from NMH by reviewing the blood pressure trends and associated symptoms and signs. In NMH, the fall in blood pressure (BP) is sudden and often is accompanied by a decrease in heart rate (HR). In OH the fall in BP is more gradual and often is accompanied by an attenuated increase in HR.

STARS IN THE DYSAUTONOMIAS UNIVERSE

There are a multitude of conditions in each age group of the dysautonomias universe. This section introduces the most common stars in that universe.

Pediatric/Inherited Dysautonomias

Several inherited or congenital diseases feature a form of dysautonomia. The following discussion describes some of them. Most are severe and become manifest in infancy or childhood.

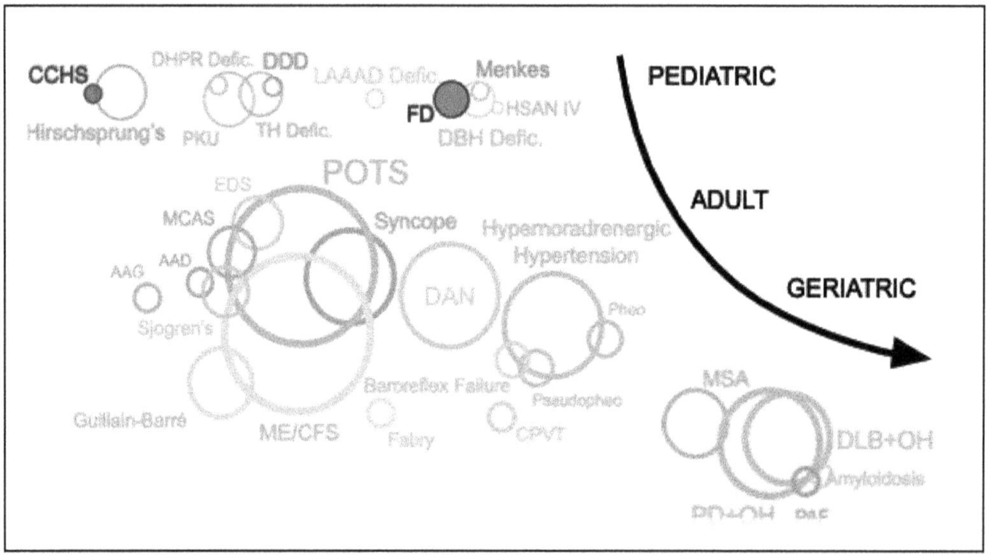

Pediatric inherited forms of dysautonomia are rare but can be severe or lethal.

Hereditary sensory and autonomic neuropathies (HSANs)

HSANs are a family of inherited conditions that all feature decreased ability to sense pain. Because of the sensory loss, the patients can self-mutilate. All forms of HSAN are rare. The most common is familial dysautonomia (HSAN III).

Familial dysautonomia (FD)

The most well-known inherited dysautonomia is familial dysautonomia (FD), also known as Riley-Day syndrome and hereditary sensory and autonomic neuropathy type III (HSAN III). FD is a rare inherited disease that features abnormalities in sensation and in functions of the autonomic nervous system. FD runs in families of Ashkenazi extraction.

The cause of FD is a mutation of the gene, IKBKAP. The mutation results in decreased levels of the protein, IkappaB kinase-associated protein (IKAP), especially in nervous system tissue. The functions of IKAP remain unknown, but it may have something to do with the development of small nerve fibers, such as non-myelinated sensory fibers and post-ganglionic sympathetic noradrenergic nerves. With supportive treatment, the outlook for FD patients has improved greatly over recent years; many patients are over 20 years old. Children with FD have a few signs that are diagnostic, including lack of overflow tears, lack of lingual fungiform papillae, and absence of a histamine flare reaction. Adult FD patients typically have orthostatic hypotension, associated with subnormal increments in plasma levels of the sympathetic neurotransmitter, norepinephrine, when the patient stands up.

FD patients are prone to crises of vomiting, sweating, fast heart rate, and high blood pressure. The crises can be life-threatening. The patients often have severe orthopedic problems. Because of inability to sense heat, the patients are at high risk of burns of the mouth or esophagus due to drinking scalding hot liquid.

With genetic screening tests, FD can be detected in utero. FD seems to involve incomplete development of sympathetic noradrenergic nerves. Adult FD patients have neuroimaging evidence for decreased cardiac sympathetic innervation, especially in the left ventricular free wall. The ratio of DOPA/DHPG in plasma is increased in all FD patients, probably reflecting decreased norepinephrine synthesis. Over the course of the disease there is evidence for progression of the sympathetic noradrenergic denervation, as plasma DOPA/DHPG ratios increase.

FD is associated not only with decreased afferent traffic from pain sensors but also with decreased afferent traffic from baroreceptors. The afferent baroreflex failure in FD might contribute to the tendency toward crises in response to seemingly minor stressors.

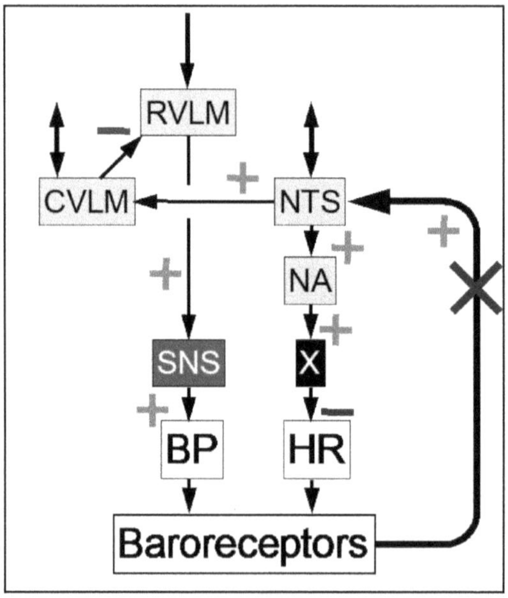

Afferent baroreflex failure in FD interferes with negative feedback loops.

Congenital central hypoventilation syndrome (CCHS)

Congenital central hypoventilation syndrome (CCHS) has been called "Ondine's curse." According to an old myth, the sea nymph Ondine ("unda" is Latin for "wave") falls in love with and marries a mortal, but he commits adultery, and as punishment he is cursed in that if he ever fell asleep he would stop breathing and die. There are other versions of the story, but it is the striking peculiarity of the curse that is sticky.

The main manifestation of CCHS is apnea (lack of breathing) during sleep. The patients breathe normally while awake, but they hypoventilate during sleep. The drop in blood oxygen tension and buildup of carbon dioxide do not stimulate ventilation.

In most cases the causative gene of CCHS is in the paired like homeobox gene (PHOX2B). Mutation in this gene is now required to diagnose CCHS. CCHS also seems to involve loss of neurons in the locus ceruleus, the main source of norepinephrine in the brain and an important center for arousal and vigilance.

CCHS is associated commonly—but not always—with manifestations of autonomic failure, including pupillary abnormalities, hypothermia, decreased sweating, decreased heart rate variability, episodes of sinus arrest, and Hirschsprung's disease.

CCHS also is associated with poor cognitive development, which may be attributed to repeated prolonged bouts of cerebral hypoxia. CCHS can now be diagnosed in neonates. Thanks to early institution of artificial ventilation, CCHS patients can now live into adulthood with better neurocognitive outcome. For more information abut pediatric dysautonomias see the full text online.

Adolescent/Adult Dysautonomias

There are many forms of dysautonomia in adolescents or adults. In general, the more common they are, the more mysterious their causes and disease mechanisms. This section summarizes the most well-know dysautonomias seen in adolescent and adult patients.

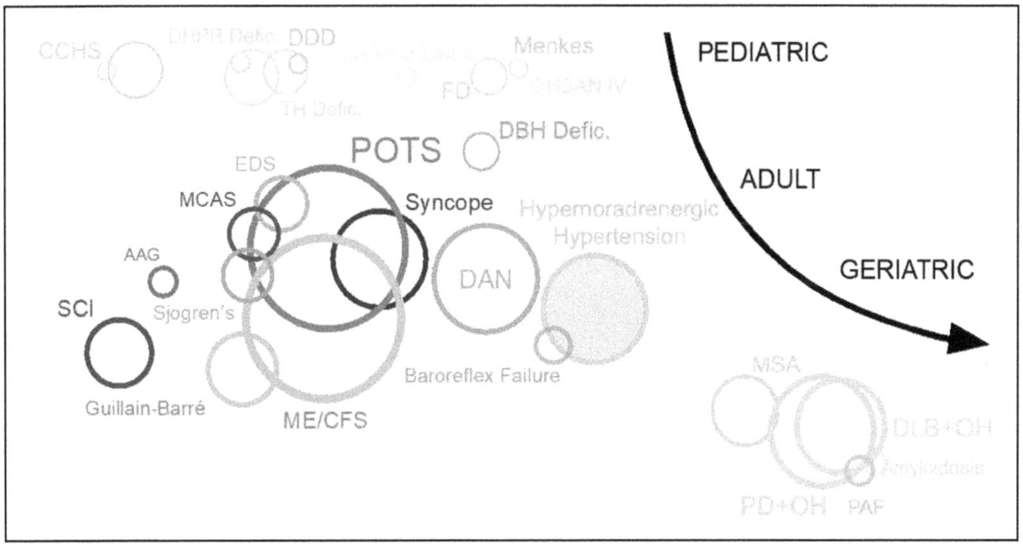

Examples of adolescent/adult dysautonomias. These often feature chronic orthostatic intolerance, an inability to tolerate prolonged standing. In the adult constellation it is more likely that there is dysfunction than degeneration of components of the autonomic nervous system.

Chronic orthostatic intolerance (COI) syndromes

In the clinical practice of adolescent/adult autonomic medicine, probably the most commonly encountered complaint is chronic orthostatic intolerance (COI), a persistent inability to tolerate standing up. This section considers two forms of COI: autonomically mediated syncope and postural tachycardia syndrome (POTS).

Autonomically mediated syncope

(Neurocardiogenic Syncope, Vasovagal Syncope, Vasodepressor Syncope or Neurally Mediated Syncope)

Syncope is sudden loss of consciousness associated with loss of muscle tone and the regaining of consciousness within seconds to minutes. In pre-syncope, the patient feels like he or she will faint but does not actually lose consciousness.

Fainting is by far the most common cause of sudden loss of consciousness in the general population. It occurs predominantly in young adults and is more common in women than in men. In elderly adults, syncope is more likely to be a sign of a heart problem (abnormal heart rhythm, abnormal conduction of electrical impulses in the heart, or heart valve problem) or orthostatic hypotension.

While there are many names used to describe this condition I use the term, autonomically mediated syncope because of the key role of alterations in activities of the components of the ANS in fainting.

Autonomically Mediated Syncope:

- Mainly young adult women or children.
- Normal pulse rate during standing.
- Decreased blood pressure during standing
- Several associated problems (inability to tolerate prolonged standing, heat intolerance, fatigue, chest pain, heart "flip- flops," brain fog, exercise intolerance).
- Variable outlook, can improve. Not life-threatening.

Many patients with frequent episodes of autonomically mediated syncope recognize early symptoms and signs of a fainting reaction coming on and are able to abort the episode before frank loss of consciousness occurs.

Patients in whom autonomically mediated syncope is a frequent problem often feel unwell between episodes, with an inability to tolerate prolonged standing, chronic fatigue, headache, "brain fog," or chest pain.

Autonomically mediated syncope can resemble POTS. Both conditions mainly involve young adult women, and both are associated with inability to tolerate prolonged standing, chronic fatigue, and headache.
As in POTS, in autonomically mediated syncope there does not seem to be much risk of later development of a chronic cardiovascular or neurodegenerative disease.

Sympathoadrenal imbalance

Increased activity of the sympathetic adrenergic system (SAS) is a characteristic feature of autonomically mediated syncope. Unfortunately, provocative tilt table testing as done in most centers rarely includes serial blood sampling for assays of plasma catecholamine levels, and this prominent finding usually is missed, despite clinical signs of SAS hyperactivity such as pallor, sweating, and pupillary dilation.

> Autonomically mediated syncope is associated with elevated plasma epinephrine levels.

Autonomically mediated syncope entails a larger increase in SAS outflow than in sympathetic noradrenergic system (SNS) outflow—"sympathoadrenal imbalance," or SAI.

The neurochemical hallmark of SAI is a proportionately greater increase in the plasma adrenaline level than in the simultaneously measured plasma norepinephrine level. This particular pattern of alterations in activities of two components of the ANS is the main reason for referring to the condition as autonomically mediated syncope.

Since SAI can precede episodes of autonomically mediated syncope, SAI may be a causal factor in fainting.

Pallor a classic sign in autonomically mediated syncope, may be due to the cutaneous vasoconstriction evoked by high circulating EPI levels. High circulating EPI levels could also explain the dilated pupils typically noted when people faint. Increased sweating often also typically precedes autonomically mediated syncope. Although this can occur at the same time as SAI, it has not yet been shown that EPI evokes the sweating. All these signs can distinguish autonomically mediated syncope from somatization, factitious syncope, and malingering.

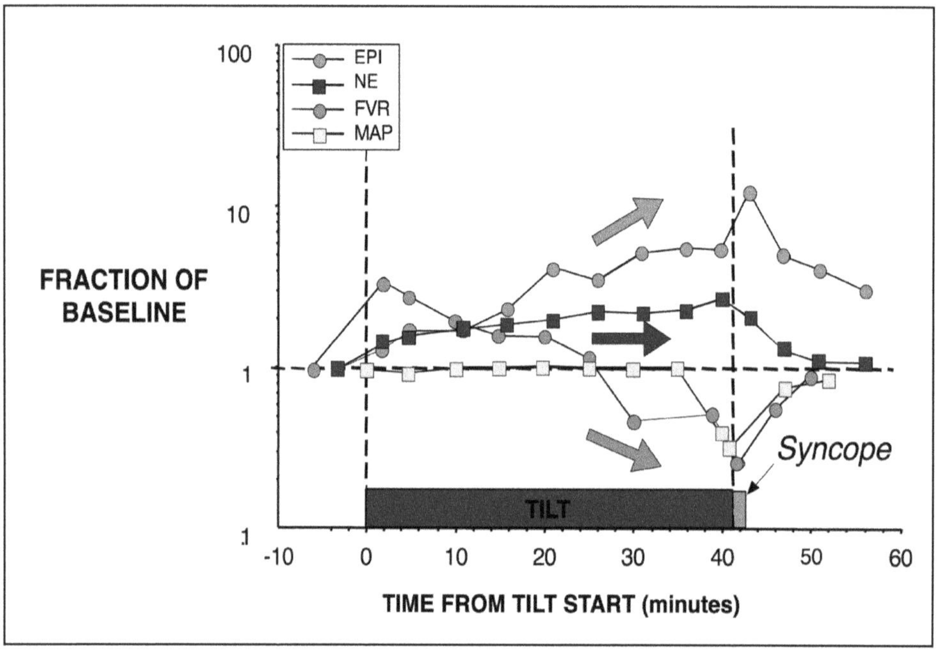

Sympathoadrenal imbalance (SAI) before tilt-evoked syncope. Plasma epinephrine (EPI) increases and forearm vascular resistance (FVR) decreases, while plasma norepinephrine (NE) remains relatively stable before the acute fall in mean arterial pressure (MAP).

Fainting in astronauts

After prolonged exposure to zero-gravity during spaceflight, returning astronauts all have orthostatic intolerance on landing day. In female astronauts the risk of syncope during head-up tilt table testing on landing day is essentially 100%.

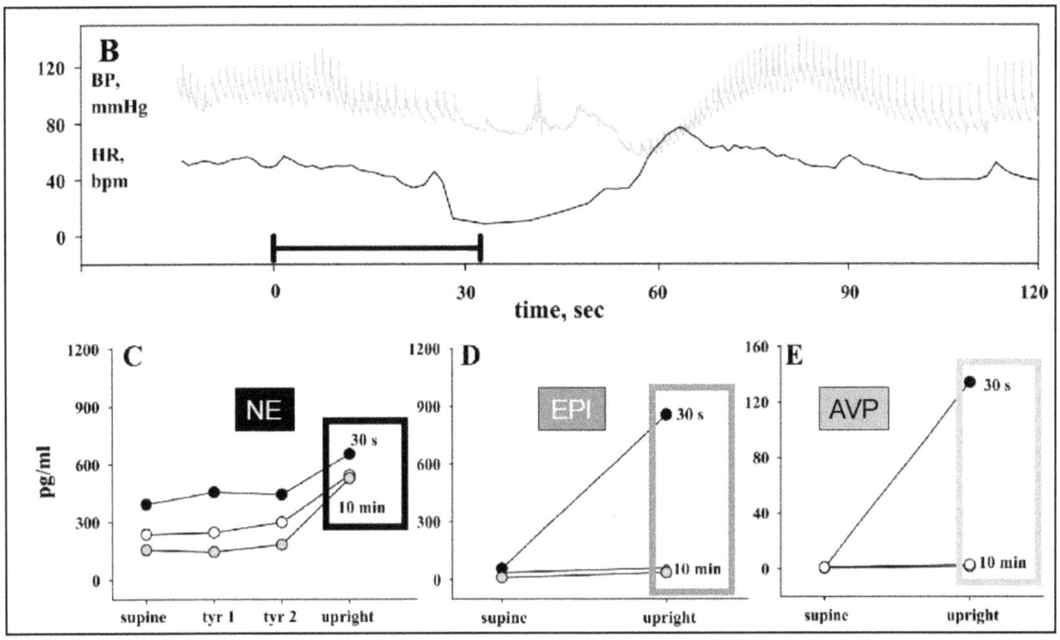

Tilt-evoked sympathoadrenal imbalance and autonomically mediated syncope in a healthy woman after prolonged exposure to zero-gravity.

The period of orthostatic intolerance in returning astronauts is quite short, in contrast to the situation in chronic orthostatic intolerance. Vigorous, frequent bouts of exercise during spaceflight and intravenous saline infusion upon return decrease the risk.

The concept diagram shows a potential mechanism of tilt-evoked autonomically-mediated syncope.

Orthostasis decreases venous return to the heart. Reflexive activation of the sympathetic noradrenergic system (SNS) tightens blood vessels, so that blood flow to the brain is maintained. In SAI there is attenuation or absence of the reflexive increase in SNS outflow, and EPI-induce skeletal muscle vasodilation is unopposed. The cardiac output is shifted away from the brain. When the individual senses there is something wrong, a distress response augments EPI release and precipitates a neurocirculatory positive feedback loop ending in critically low cerebral blood flow and loss of consciousness.

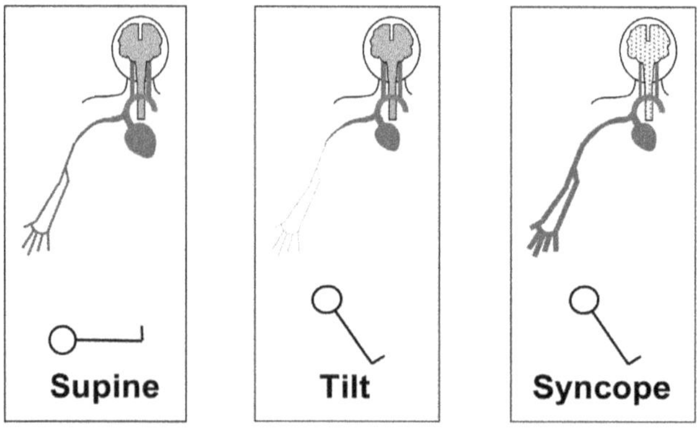

An explanation for tilt-evoked, autonomically-mediated syncope based on sympathoadrenal imbalance shunting blood toward skeletal muscle at the expense of blood flow to the brain.

Postural tachycardia syndrome (POTS)

Postural tachycardia syndrome (POTS) probably is the most common form of chronic orthostatic intolerance (COI).

In general medical practice, the finding of an excessive increase in heart rate with standing s usually secondary to identifiable problems such as medications or dehydration from chronic illness. It is only when the cause is not readily identified and the patient has some of the other complaints discussed below that the patient is thought to have POTS:

- Mainly young adult women.
- Excessive Increase in HR during standing 30 bpm adults (40 bpm teens)
- Several associated problems (chronic fatigue, exercise and heat intolerance, headache, neuropathic pain, slowed gastrointestinal movements, chest pain, heart "flip-flops," tendency to panic)
- Variable outlook, can improve. Not life-threatening. Can be disabling.

At least some of the symptoms of POTS are thought to reflect increased effects of the catecholamines norepinephrine or epinephrine, from overactivity of the sympathetic noradrenergic system (SNS), the sympathetic adrenergic system (SAS), or both. Cardiac norepinephrine spillover is increased in POTS patients even while they are supine.

The key to POTS is the "S"

The key word in postural tachycardia syndrome is not "tachycardia" but "syndrome." POTS is a syndrome, not a disease. A syndrome is a set of symptoms that occur together. Merely having a fast pulse rate while standing is not a syndrome. POTS always involves more than orthostatic tachycardia alone.

Patients with POTS always have several symptoms, such as orthostatic intolerance, "brain fog," exercise intolerance, chronic fatigue, a tendency to faint, chest pain, pain in the back of the neck or shoulders ("coat hanger phenomenon"), headache, cool, sweaty extremities, heat intolerance, palpitations, gastrointestinal complaints (nausea, early satiety, slow gastrointestinal transit, bloating, gastroesophageal reflux, abdominal pain), delayed orthostatic syncope, disturbed sleep, panic, anxiety, depression, and generalized disability.

> The occurrence of a rapid pulse rate when a person stands is necessary but is not sufficient to diagnose POTS.

Researchers have thought that usually in POTS, sympathetic nerve traffic to the heart is increased as a form of compensatory activation. The possibility of blood volume depletion or excessive pooling of blood in the legs during standing up has drawn particular attention. Indeed, low blood volume was noted in the first reported case of POTS.

Dehydration, blood loss, or other causes of decreased blood volume can produce a condition that looks like POTS. Low blood volume in turn can result from blood loss, from failure of the bone marrow to produce an adequate number of red blood cells, or from failure of hormone systems such as the renin-angiotensin-aldosterone system.

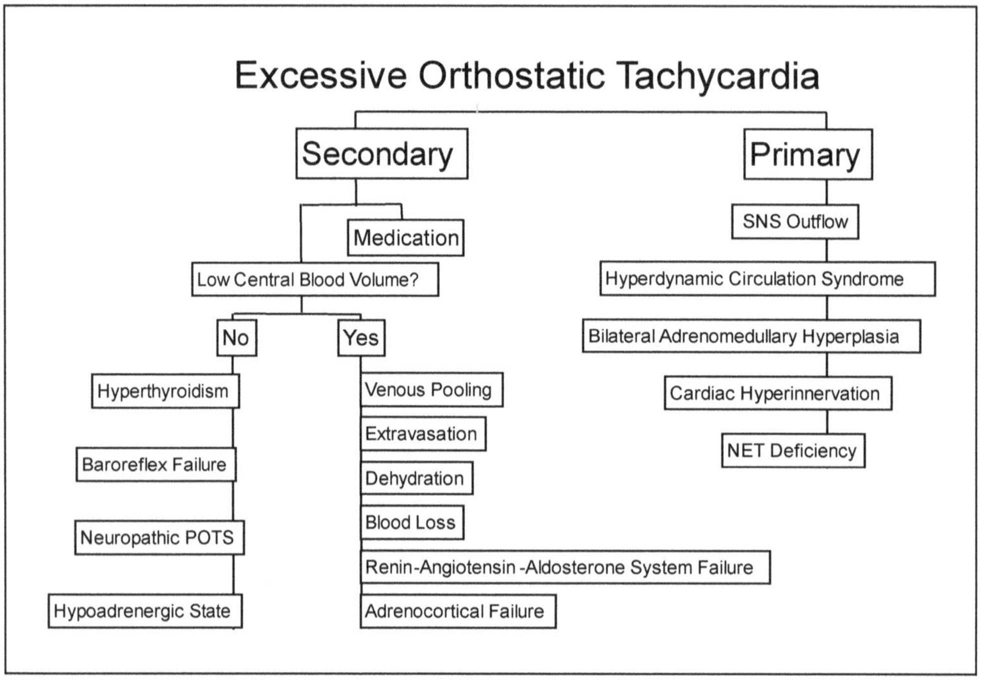

Excessive orthostatic tachycardia, the defining characteristic of postural tachycardia syndrome (POTS), has many potential causes. They can be divided in terms of secondary or primary determinants of increased cardiac sympathetic outflow during orthostasis.

An "effective" low blood volume can occur, when the blood pools excessively in the veins in the pelvis and abdomen after a person stands. Consistent with the blood pooling idea, inflation of a military anti-shock trousers (MAST) suit reduces substantially the increase in heart rate in response to orthostasis in patients with POTS.

An excessive shift in blood volume distribution might reflect a lack of muscular "tone" in the vein walls. For instance, a problem with the protein structure of blood vessel walls could lead to POTS in Ehlers-Danlos syndrome.

POTS patients often have high plasma levels of norepinephrine (NE) when they are standing up. According to one suggestion, criteria for diagnosing POTS include an upright plasma NE level of 600 pg/mL or more; however, whether increased SNS outflows constitute a primary abnormality or compensatory response usually is unknown in an individual patient.

In a related syndrome called the hyperdynamic circulation syndrome the patients have a fast pulse rate independently of posture, labile hypertension, increased heart rate responses to the beta-adrenoceptor agonist isoproterenol, and increased plasma NE and adrenaline levels both at rest and during provocative maneuvers. Beta-adrenoceptor blockers such as propranolol or benzodiazepines such as diazepam improve the symptoms. It is unclear whether patients with hyperdynamic circulation syndrome have an increased frequency of later development of established hypertension. Episodes of fast pulse rate and increased blood pressure can be associated with blotchy flushing of the face, neck, and upper chest.

POTS can result from mutation of the gene that encodes the cell membrane norepinephrine transporter (NET). POTS from this genetic cause is very rare.

In "neuropathic POTS," sympathetic nerves to the heart are thought to be overactive as a compensation for loss of sympathetic nerves elsewhere.

Although POTS and autonomically mediated syncope (neurocardiogenic syncope, vasovagal syncope, frequent fainting) are considered to be different forms of chronic orthostatic intolerance, when POTS patients are subjected to tilt table testing a substantial minority have tilt-evoked hypotension. When they do they have the same pattern of sympathoadrenal imbalance (SAI) as found in patients with fainting who do not have POTS.

Mast cell activation syndrome (MCAS)

Mast cells are a type of immune cell that plays a key role in acute allergic responses. They express receptors for IgE, the immune globulin involved with anaphylaxis, as well as receptors for a variety of other chemical messengers.

When activated, mast cells release several compounds, including monoamines such as histamine, serotonin, and dopamine, as well as cytokines such as TNF-α, interleukins, prostaglandins, and leukotrienes. Taken together these compounds exert important effects on the cardiovascular, respiratory, and gastrointestinal systems and the skin.

In Mast Cell Activation Syndrome (MCAS), the mast cells release their chemicals inappropriately or excessively.

Symptoms of MCAS include flushing, itching, diarrhea, nausea, wheezing, fatigue, "brain fog," orthostatic intolerance, and fainting reactions.

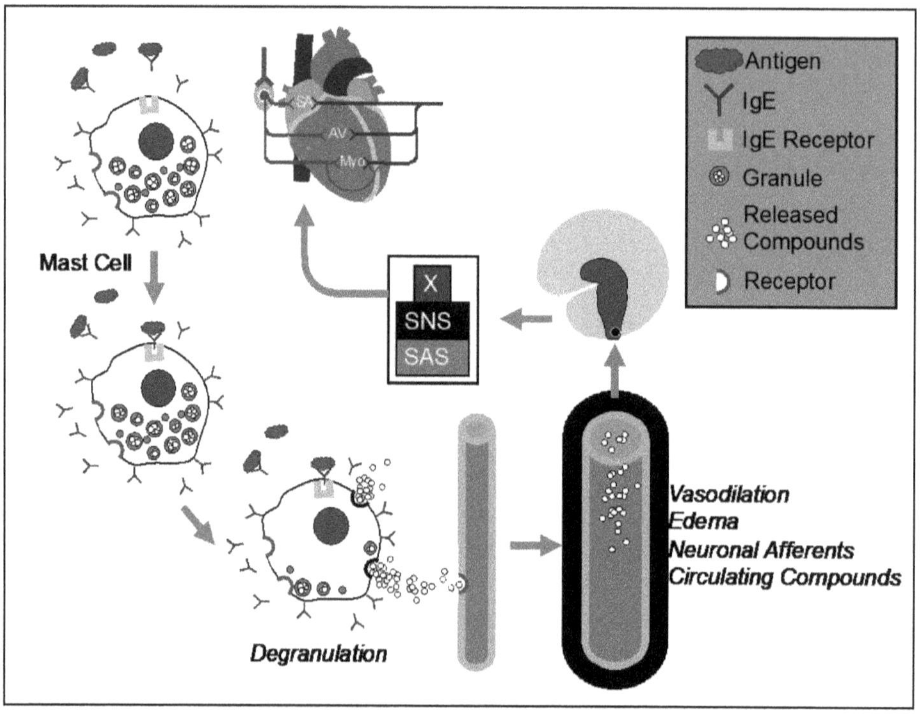

Concept diagram illustrating how mast cell activation could produce orthostatic intolerance and excessive orthostatic tachycardia.

To determine whether a patient with orthostatic intolerance has MCAS, it has been proposed that three criteria should be met:

1. The patient should have symptoms consistent with MCAS, such as repeated episodes of flushing, itching, nasal congestion, coughing, chest tightness, wheezing, abdominal pain, or diarrhea.
2. There should be laboratory evidence of mast cell activation.
3. There should be improvement of symptoms with the use of medications such as anti-histamines or leukotriene receptor blockers. Cromolyn sodium, which stabilizes mast cells, is also used. Although patients with Mast Cell Activation Syndrome (MCAS) often have symptoms of POTS, the frequency of MCAS in POTS is unknown.

MCAS, Ehlers-Danlos syndrome, and POTS can occur together. The bases for this triad are poorly understood.

Baroreflex failure

Uncommonly, chronic orthostatic intolerance reflects baroreflex failure. In this situation the sympathetic noradrenergic system is not activated appropriately in response to a decrease in blood pressure or to a decrease in venous return to the heart. Baroreflex failure does not consistently cause orthostatic hypotension, but it always causes large swings in blood pressure, both high and low, because of the inability to keep the blood pressure within limits.

Baroreflex failure occurs in some people years after irradiation of the neck, such as for treating a cancer. The radioactivity exposure accelerates aging-related stiffness of the carotid arteries in the neck—arteriosclerosis. Since the baroreceptors are distortion receptors, the stiffening interferes with the ability of the baroreceptors to sense changes in blood pressure.

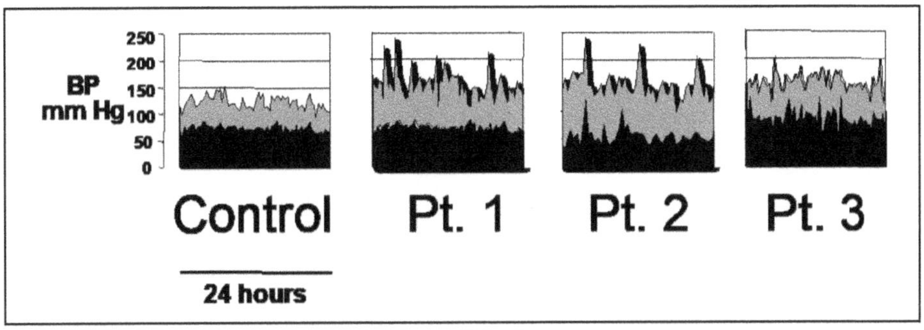

Increased 24-hour blood pressure variability in patients with baroreflex failure as a late sequela of neck irradiation.

Baroreflex failure is also a known complication of tumors and surgery for tumors in the lower brainstem, the location of the "barostat" for blood pressure regulation.

Spinal cord injury (SCI)

The vagus nerve is derived from the brainstem, which would be above the level of spinal cord transection. Spinal cord injury (SCI) disrupts the pathways descending from the central autonomic network to the sympathetic and the sacral parasympathetic nerves.

In patients with spinal cord transection, the nervous connections between the autonomic pre-ganglionic neurons in the intermediolateral columns of the spinal cord and the ganglia and post-ganglionic neurons remain intact. This sets the stage for a phenomenon called "autonomic dysreflexia."

When the urinary bladder (or the rectum) is distended, sympathetic noradrenergic outflow to the cardiovascular system increases via a spinal reflex. Because of the disruption of the baroreflexes, there is no buffering of the increase in blood pressure.

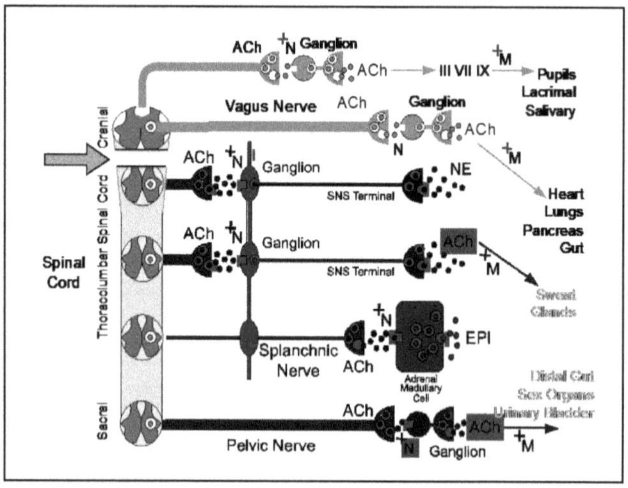

In spinal cord injury there is a disruption of descending nerve fibers of the sympathetic noradrenergic system (SNS), while parasympathetic innervation of the head and vagal outflow to the heart are intact.

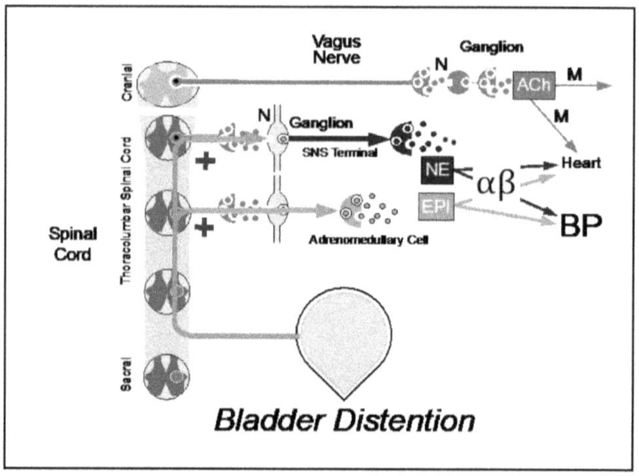

In autonomic dysreflexia, distention of the bladder or rectum increases the blood pressure (BP), probably via release of norepinephrine (NE) from sympathetic nerves and epinephrine (EPI) from the adrenal medulla.

In patients with SCI the nervous connections between the autonomic pre-ganglionic neurons in the intermediolateral columns of the spinal cord and the ganglia and post-ganglionic neurons remain intact. This sets the stage for a phenomenon called "autonomic dysreflexia.

When the urinary bladder (or the rectum) is distended, sympathetic noradrenergic outflow to the cardiovascular system increases via a spinal reflex. Because of the disruption of the baroreflexes, there is no buffering of the increase in blood pressure.

Dopamine-beta-hydroxylase (DBH) deficiency

DBH deficiency constitutes a rare cause of SNS failure due to the inability to synthesize norepinephrine (NE). Because of isolated noradrenergic deficiency, sympathetic cholinergic function is intact, and DBH-deficient patients therefore sweat normally when exposed to heat, even though they have severe orthostatic hypotension due to SNS failure. (Actually, SNS nerve traffic is unimpaired in DBH deficiency, but instead of NE being released it is dopamine that is released from the nerve terminals.)

Immunity-associated dysautonomias

There are a variety of dysautonomias for which links with immunological problems have been described. This is a rapidly expanding area in autonomic medicine in adolescents and adults. Some clinicians have tried intravenous immunoglobulin (IVIG) to treat patients who have acute or subacute onset of POTS or autonomically mediated syncope.

Sjogren's syndrome is an autoimmune condition in which the patients have chronically dry mouth and dry eyes, typically in the setting of some form of connective tissue disease like rheumatoid arthritis. There is evidence of autoimmunity directed against the salivary glands and lacrimal glands, with infiltration of the tissue by lymphocytes.

The vast majority of Sjogren's syndrome patients are adult women—just as is the case for POTS, autonomically mediated syncope, chronic fatigue syndrome, temporomandibular joint disorder, and migraine. One of the most famous patients with the condition is the professional tennis player, Venus Williams. She has suffered for years with chronic fatigue that accompanies her Sjogren's syndrome. Since having to drop out of the US Open in 2011, she has returned to close to her former performance, with a vegan diet and exercise regimen.

Sjogren's syndrome has long been suspected of involving a form of dysautonomia. A report suggested dysfunction of the parasympathetic nervous system (PNS); however, sympathetic noradrenergic system (SNS) function seems intact.

Guillain-Barré syndrome is a condition in which there is autoimmune attack on peripheral nerves. The syndrome often follows by a few days or weeks after a respiratory or gastrointestinal viral infection or surgery. The target tissue is the myelin sheath surrounding nerves or the nerve fibers themselves. The longer nerves are affected earlier, explaining initial findings in the feet or hands, with a centripetal progression. The symptoms and signs are of an ascending symmetric weakness or paralysis and altered sensation beginning in the feet and moving upwards in the body. The patient's clinical status declines over the course of hours to weeks, with the condition at its worst after a few weeks. In severe cases the patient becomes totally paralyzed and can die from respiratory failure. Eventually the patient recovers, although there can be residual weakness.

Guillain-Barré syndrome patients can develop a form of reversible heart failure that may be mediated by catecholamines. The condition resembles takotsubo cardiopathy.

Autoimmune Autonomic Ganglionopathy (AAG): The lady who couldn't spit

Several years ago, at the NIH Clinical Center I evaluated an elderly African-American resident of the District of Columbia for severe orthostatic hypotension. She did have orthostatic intolerance, but this was not her chief complaint. Her chief complaint was that she couldn't make spit.

Her mouth was so dry, she couldn't chew food. She was also severely constipated. The combination of not being able to salivate and having severe constipation had resulted in her becoming malnourished. When I first saw her, she looked cachexic, like a concentration camp survivor or a patient with end-stage cancer.

She had characteristic abnormalities of beat-to-beat blood pressure associated with the Valsalva maneuver, indicating that her orthostatic hypotension was not from dehydration but from a neurogenic cause. She also had an extremely low plasma norepinephrine level. Initially I thought she had pure autonomic failure (PAF), and I predicted that her 18F-dopamine PET scan would show loss of sympathetic innervation of the heart. Instead, her 18F-dopamine scan was normal. Under the study protocol she received a ganglion blocker, and this produced hardly any effects at all.

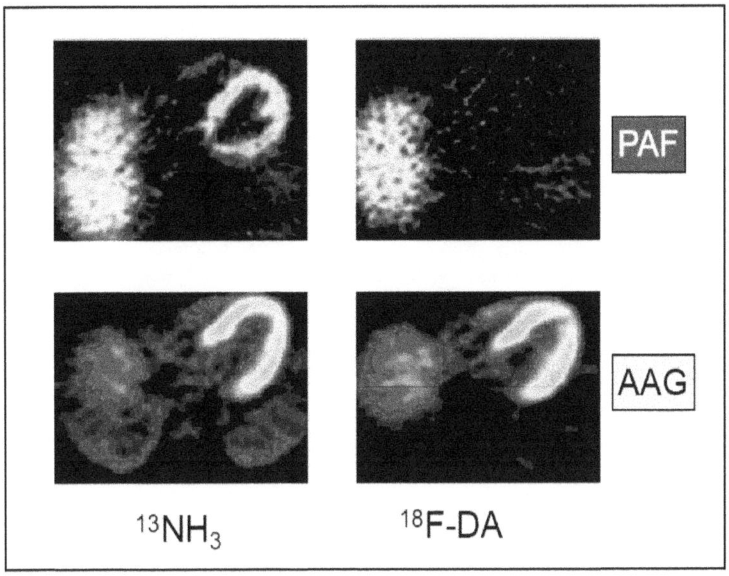

Intact cardiac sympathetic innervation in autoimmune autonomic ganglionopathy.

At about that time Dr. Steven Vernino (then at the Mayo Clinic) had published a study about autoimmune autonomic neuropathy associated with a circulating antibody to the neuronal nicotinic receptor, which mediates ganglionic neurotransmission. No patient with PAF had had such an antibody; I suspected our patient might and sent Dr. Vernino a sample, which was positive. Together we published the first case of what has come to be known as autoimmune autonomic ganglionopathy (AAG). AAG is a quite a rare form of acquired autonomic failure in which there is decreased activity of all the components of the autonomic nervous system—pandysautonomia.

Amyloidosis

Amyloidosis refers to a variety of disorders that have in common deposition of a mis-folded protein called amyloid in body organs. Normally the protein is soluble, but the misfolding causes the protein to precipitate. The disease manifestations depend on the organs involved—especially the heart and kidneys.

Amyloidosis can involve the sensory and autonomic fibers in peripheral nerves. Peripheral neuropathy in amyloidosis is usually symmetrical. I remember a case of amyloid-associated autonomic failure where the patient wore gloves continuously, even in his hospital bed at the NIH Clinical Center, in an effort to decrease his distressing "pins and needles" sensations.

One can diagnose amyloidosis by biopsying mucous membranes (rectal, buccal) or abdominal fat pad tissue and looking under a microscope for deposits of the amyloid material. Congo red staining, especially when combined with polarized light, demonstrates the proteins microscopically.

Patients with amyloidosis can have a marked reduction of myocardial noradrenergic nerves, as indicated by cardiac sympathetic neuroimaging.

Diabetic autonomic neuropathy

Diabetes is probably the most common cause of autonomic neuropathy. Among patients with diabetes, the occurrence of autonomic neuropathy is an adverse prognostic factor.

Diabetes often involves chronic pain in the feet (painful diabetic neuropathy). Loss of sympathetic noradrenergic innervation in the feet accompanies the neuropathy.

Diabetics can also have neurogenic orthostatic hypotension, with evidence of failure of baroreflex regulation of sympathetic noradrenergic system outflows.

Poor control of the urinary bladder is another sign of diabetic autonomic neuropathy. Patients have difficulty starting the urinary stream or have urinary retention that can require self- catheterization.

Other manifestations of diabetic autonomic neuropathy include erectile dysfunction, resting tachycardia, diarrhea or constipation, esophageal dysfunction, and decreased stomach contractions (gastroparesis).

The high prevalence, multiple manifestations, and prognostic significance of diabetic autonomic neuropathy contrast with remarkably poor understanding of the mechanisms.

Geriatric Dysautonomias

Geriatric dysautonomias can result from degenerative processes in the central autonomic network or in autonomic nerves supplying body organs. Many of these conditions are characterized by misfolding and abnormal deposition of proteins, such as alpha-synuclein (αS), amyloid, and tau.

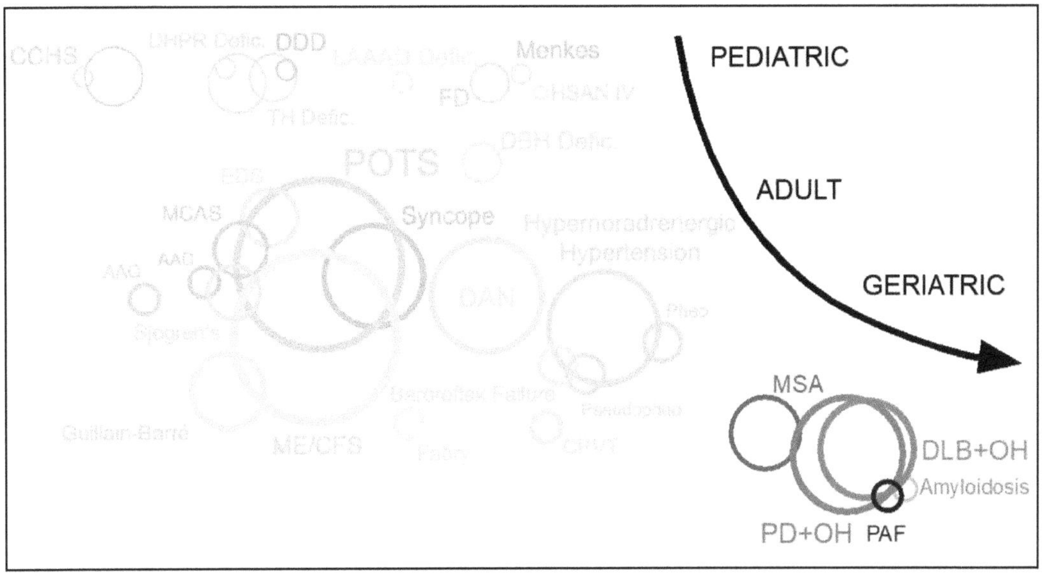

Dysautonomias in the elderly often reflect degeneration of components of the autonomic nervous system.

Autonomic synucleinopathies

Neurologists have recognized three forms of "primary" chronic autonomic failure—pure autonomic failure (PAF), multiple system atrophy (MSA), and autonomic failure in the setting of Parkinson's disease (PD). Now it is known that all three conditions come under the umbrella of "synucleinopathies," meaning that they all involve abnormal deposits of αS.

The αS story is relatively new. In 1997 an international team of researchers reported the first identification of a genetic cause of PD—mutation of the gene encoding αS—in a rare Greek-Italian-American family in which PD was transmitted as an autosomal dominant trait, meaning that one-half of the family members, whether men or women, had PD and one-half didn't. This was an important scientific discovery, but since only one family was involved, it was unclear whether the new information would apply to PD as a whole. In the same year, however, it was found that Lewy bodies, a pathologic hallmark of PD, contain abundant precipitated αS. That is, even sporadic PD was found to involve an abnormality of αS.

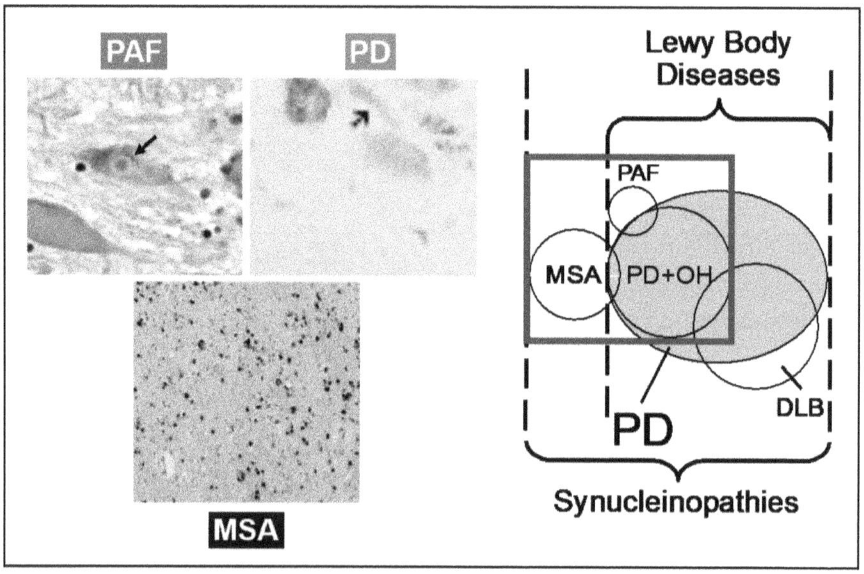

Synucleinopathies are characterized by deposition of the protein alpha-synuclein (αS) inside cells. In Lewy body forms of synucleinpathy the αS in neurons (especially catecholaminergic neurons) is in the brainstem. In multiple system atrophy (MSA) αS is in the cytoplasm of glial cells (glial cytoplasmic inclusions).

Multiple system atrophy (MSA) is also characterized by αS deposits. In MSA, the deposits are in the cytoplasm of glial cells, which are "helper" cells in the brain that are not neurons. A microscopic feature of MSA is glial cytoplasmic inclusions, or GCIs.

A major form of pure autonomic failure (PAF) also involves Lewy bodies, both in the brainstem and in sympathetic ganglia. PAF and MSA, which previously were considered to be "primary chronic autonomic failure" syndromes, are now considered to be in a family of autonomic synucleinopathies.

About 30-40% of patients with Parkinson's disease have orthostatic hypotension (OH), a fall in blood pressure every time they stand up. This subgroup has been designated "PD+OH." A substantial proportion of PD patients have dementia—PD+D, which overlaps with dementia with Lewy bodies (DLB), or Lewy body ementia. PAF, PD+OH, and DLB+OH come under the heading of Lewy body forms of neurogenic OH.

In the evaluation of a patient referred for orthostatic hypotension and possible autonomic synucleinopathy, I use a 4-step algorithm.

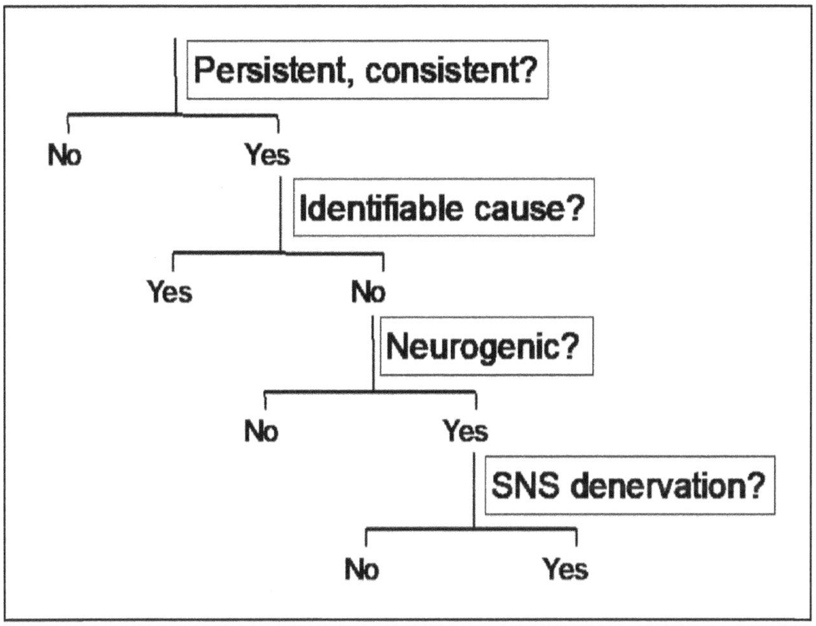

4-Step algorithm for clinical and laboratory workup of orthostatic hypotension.

First, in autonomic synucleinopathies orthostatic hypotension is a persistent, consistent finding. The patient may not always have symptoms of low blood pressure while standing, but the blood pressure always falls.

Second, secondary causes of OH such as drugs and diabetes must be excluded.

Third, the OH should be confirmed to be neurogenic. One way to do this is by assessing the beat-to-beat blood pressure responses to the Valsalva maneuver.

Fourth is to test for loss of sympathetic noradrenergic nerves. This may be done by conducting cardiac sympathetic neuroimaging, assaying plasma catechols, using neuropharmacological probes, or examining skin biopsies for loss of innervation in pilomotor muscles or in blood vessel walls. Cardiac sympathetic neuroimaging is probably most sensitive.

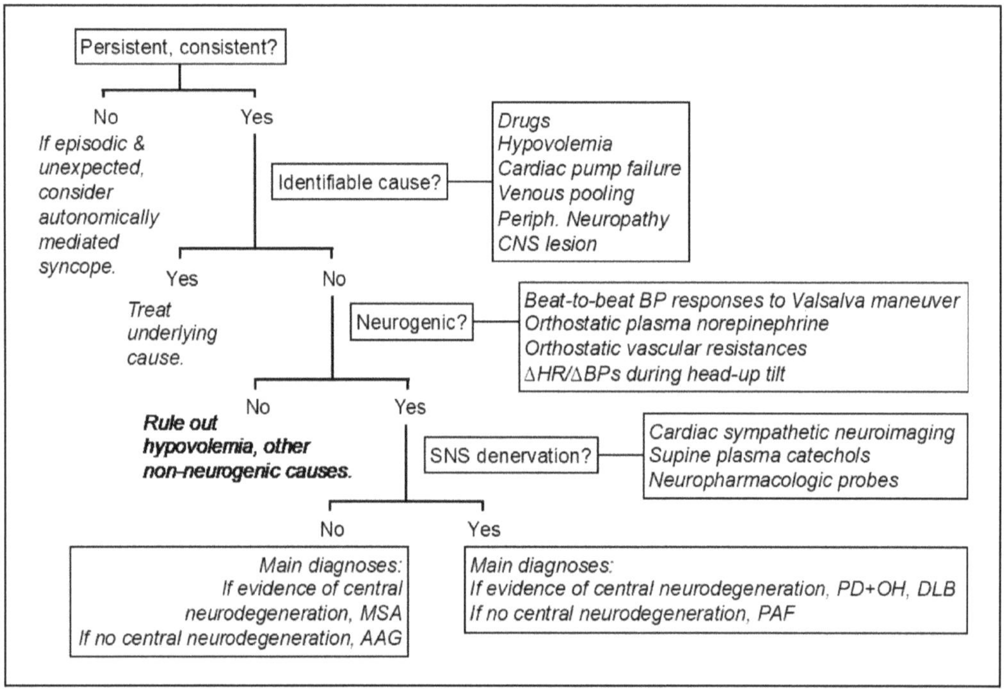

A more detailed algorithm for workup of nOH.

Autonomic synucleinopathies share two core features.

First, patients with autonomic synucleinopathy have "baroreflex-sympathoneural failure." That is, they have failure of regulation of the sympathetic noradrenergic system by the arterial baroreflex. When they perform the Valsalva maneuver, they have abnormal beat-to-beat blood pressure responses in Phases II and IV. During orthostasis their plasma norepinephrine (NE) levels increase by less than 60%, whereas in healthy people plasma NE levels approximately double within 5 minutes.

Second, autonomic synucleinopathies all involve catecholamine deficiency, in the brain, periphery, or both. Cerebrospinal fluid (CSF) levels of DOPAC, the main neuronal metabolite of dopamine, and DHPG, the main neuronal metabolite of norepinephrine, are low in PD, MSA, and PAF.

Results of cardiac sympathetic neuroimaging fit with the view that cardiac noradrenergic deficiency is a characteristic feature of Lewy body forms of autonomic synucleinopathies, in contrast with intact sympathetic noradrenergic innervation in most MSA patients. All PD+OH patients have evidence for cardiac noradrenergic deficiency, whereas most patients with MSA have intact sympathetic noradrenergic innervation. A minority of MSA patients do have evidence for a loss of cardiac sympathetic nerves; however, the finding of normal cardiac sympathetic innervation excludes PD+OH.

Another valuable clinical laboratory test in the differential diagnosis of PD+OH vs. MSA is assessment of the sense of smell, such as by the University of Pennsylvania Smell Identification Test (UPSIT). Most patients with PD+OH are anosmic. That is, the UPSIT score is 18 or less out of 40. Combining smell testing with cardiac sympathetic neuroimaging can help separate Lewy body from non-Lewy body forms of nOH.

In contrast, many MSA-P patients have normal or only slightly to moderately decreased sense of smell. In a patient with parkinsonism and neurogenic orthostatic hypotension, the finding of normal sense of smell on the UPSIT favors a diagnosis of MSA-P over PD+OH.

Pure autonomic Failure (PAF)

Pure autonomic failure (PAF) is a rare disease that features persistent falls in blood pressure when the patient stands—orthostatic hypotension (OH)—in the absence of signs of central nervous system disease and in the absence of other known causes of OH. The OH results from sympathetic neurocirculatory failure and therefore is neurogenic (nOH).

PAF patients report progressively worsening dizziness when standing up, after a large meal, upon exposure to environmental heat, or after exercise. The patients often learn to sit or stand with their legs twisted pretzel-like, since this decreases pooling of blood in the legs. In men, erectile failure is an early symptom. Often the patients have decreased sweating.

Blood pressure responses to the Valsalva maneuver in PAF always show the abnormal pattern that indicates baroreflex- sympathoneural failure. Virtually all patients with PAF have neuroimaging evidence of cardiac noradrenergic deficiency.

Because of "denervation supersensitivity" and baroreflex- sympathoneural failure, patients with PAF can have surprisingly large increases in blood pressure in response to adrenoceptor-stimulating drugs.

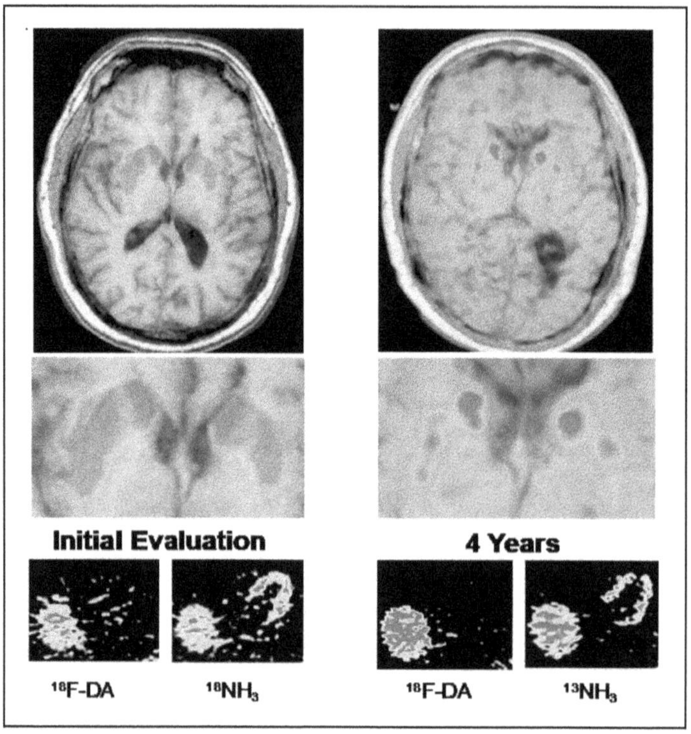

In this patient PAF evolved to dementia with Lewy bodies and pre-terminal PD.

Plasma norepinephrine (NE) levels often (but not always) are low in PAF. Because of the baroreflex-sympathoneural failure, the plasma NE level fails to increase appropriately (by ≥ 60%) when the patient stands. PAF patients usually (but not always) also have low plasma levels of 3,4-dihydroxyphenylglycol (DHPG), which is the main intra-neuronal metabolite of NE.

While chronic and causing disability, PAF is not thought to be lethal. At least in some patients, however, PAF evolves into dementia with Lewy bodies and orthostatic hypotension (DLB+OH), to Parkinson's disease with orthostatic hypotension (PD+OH).

Parkinson's disease (PD)

Parkinson's disease (or Parkinson disease, PD) is the second most common neurodegenerative disease of the elderly (the first is Alzheimer's disease). PD is well known to be characterized by a movement disorder that includes slowness (bradykinesia), limb rigidity, tremor at rest, and imbalance. The key gross anatomic change in the brain in PD is a loss of black pigmentation in the substantia nigra (from the Latin for "black substance") in the midbrain of the brainstem. The loss of black pigment probably reflects a decreased number of neurons that contain the catecholamine dopamine. It is no coincidence that dopamine in solution spontaneously oxidizes and polymerizes to form a black pigment.

A disease with no heart

The discovery of loss of cardiac sympathetic nerves in PD provided clear evidence that PD is more than a brain disease and more than a movement disorder. It is also a disease that involves loss of sympathetic noradrenergic nerves and a form of dysautonomia.

Neuroimaging evidence of cardiac noradrenergic deficiency occurs in most patients with PD and in all patients with PD with orthostatic hypotension (PD+OH).

Sympathetic noradrenergic denervation was the first identified mechanism for a non-motor aspect of PD. One would guess that the cardiac noradrenergic deficiency causes fatigue or shortness of breath during exercise.

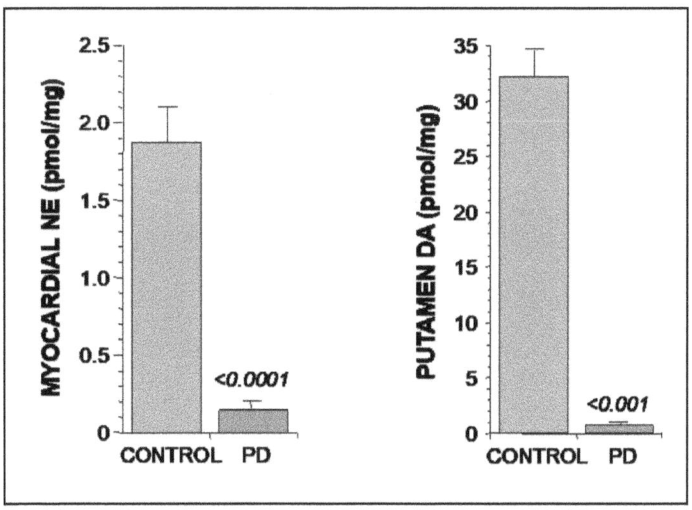

In PD there is just as severe loss of norepinephrine (NE) in the left ventricular myocardium as there is loss of dopamine (DA) in the putamen.

In PD when does cardiac sympathetic denervation develop?

The findings in a case we reported several years ago demonstrate that cardiac sympathetic denervation can precede the movement disorder by several years. This finding fits with Heiko Braak's concept about the pathogenetic sequence of synucleinopathy in PD. According to Braak there is early autonomic involvement, followed by alpha-synuclein deposition in the dorsal motor nucleus of the vagus nerve in the caudal medulla (stage 1), then in the rostral ventrolateral medulla, midline raphe nuclei, and pontine locus ceruleus (stage 2), and only in stage 3 in midbrain substantia nigra.

The patient underwent a workup at the NIH Clinical Center for a possible pheochromocytoma, a tumor that produces and releases catecholamines, because he had variable high blood pressure. As part of the testing the patient had a 18F-dopamine PET scan. The workup was negative, and he was given a diagnosis of "pseudopheochromocytoma." About 4 years later he returned for testing, this time to be in a study about pseudopheochromocytoma. He reported that over the past few months he had noted the gradual onset of slow movement, limb rigidity, a shuffling gait, and decreased facial expression.

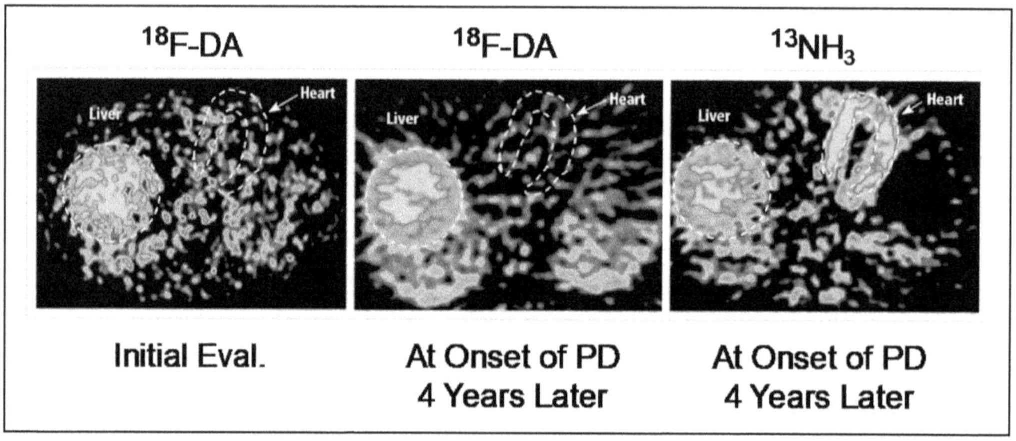

Neuroimaging evidence of cardiac noradrenergic deficiency can precede the motor onset of Parkinson's disease.

He said he felt and looked like a robot. He was diagnosed with PD by a neurology consultant. Cardiac sympathetic neuroimaging by ^{18}F-dopamine PET scanning showed a loss of sympathetic noradrenergic innervation, as is typical of PD.

In retrospect, the ^{18}F-dopamine PET scan from 4 years previously had shown the same loss of sympathetic innervation throughout the left ventricular myocardium.

This was the first reported case of cardiac sympathetic denervation preceding motor signs of PD.

On the other hand, patients who already have symptomatic PD can have normal or only localized loss of cardiac sympathetic innervation. This doesn't fit with Braak's concept. For instance, in a who already had PD, cardiac sympathetic innervation seemed normal over about 8 years of follow-up. Then the patient developed partial denervation in the left ventricular free wall. This was followed soon after by diffuse denervation, with loss of innervation in the inter-ventricular septum.

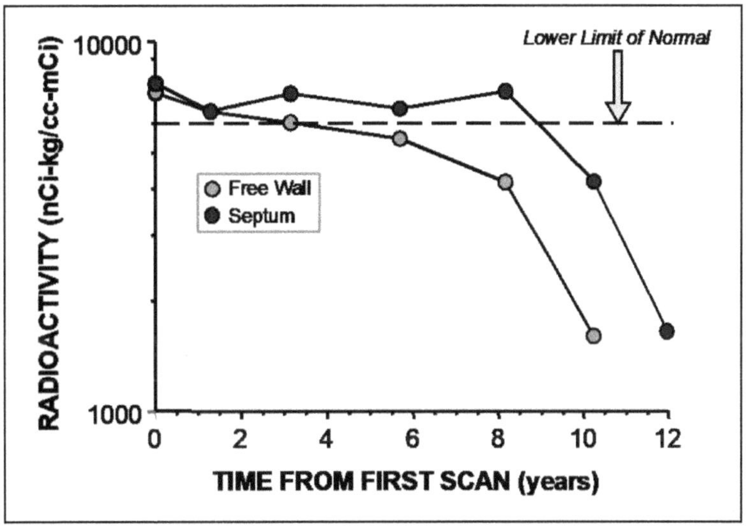

Neuroimaging evidence for loss of cardiac sympathetic innervation can be a late finding in patients who already have PD.

Across patients with PD there is no relationship between the extent of the putamen dopaminergic lesion, as indicated by the putamen/occipital cortex ratio of 18F-DOPA-derived radioactivity, and the extent of the sympathetic noradrenergic lesion, as indicated by the septal myocardial concentration of 18F-dopamine-derived radioactivity. Instead, the loss of cardiac sympathetic noradrenergic nerves seems to occur independently of the striatal dopaminergic lesion underlying the movement disorder.

In some patients the finding of cardiac sympathetic denervation might be a biomarker predicting later development of PD, while in others cardiac sympathetic denervation is a late finding. It seems that all PD patients eventually lose cardiac sympathetic nerves. It may take several years for this to begin, but once it does, the loss progresses rapidly.

PD with orthostatic hypotension (PD+OH)

Symptoms or signs of autonomic dysfunction occur extremely commonly in PD. These include constipation, urinary frequency and urgency, drooling, erectile failure in men, altered sweating, and orthostatic intolerance due to orthostatic hypotension.

Exactly how these problems, which reflect involvement of different components of the autonomic nervous system, relate to each other is unclear. For instance, in PD the prevalence of constipation and urinary frequency and urgency is about the same regardless of the occurrence of orthostatic hypotension (OH).

The frequency of OH is underestimated when clinicians depend on symptoms or signs, because many patients with OH feel nothing wrong when they are upright or have symptoms that are non-specific.

Orthostatic hypotension (OH) in PD is always associated with evidence of sympathetic noradrenergic deficiency. In contrast, sweat production, which is mainly a function of the sympathetic cholinergic system, can be normal in PD+OH, and the majority of PD+OH patients have normal QSART results. This means that the sympathetic lesion in PD+OH is neurotransmitter-specific. The results of cardiac sympathetic neuroimaging are so consistent that in a patient with parkinsonism and OH the finding of normal cardiac sympathetic innervation excludes PD+OH.

Patients with PD often have constipation and urinary urgency, frequency, and incontinence. These might reflect a form of failure of the parasympathetic nervous system (PNS); whether this is the case remains unknown. Decreased traffic in the vagus nerve, the nerve of the PNS that supplies the heart, appears to cause the constant pulse rate seen in most patients with PD+OH. This could reflect a loss of parasympathetic nerves or a problem in reflexive regulation of traffic in intact nerves.

The long-term outlook in PD+OH is worse than in PD without OH (PD No OH). When the movement disorder first becomes apparent, PD+OH patients are on average about a decade older than PD No OH patients. Even after adjustment for age, however, PD+OH patients have shorter survival than do PD No OH patients.

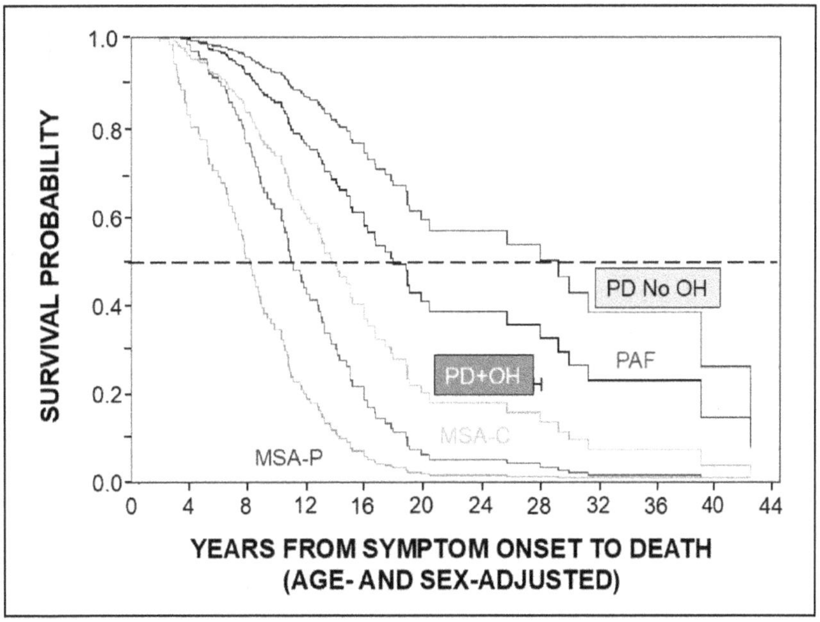

In PD the occurrence of OH shortens survival.

Multiple system atrophy (MSA)

Multiple system atrophy ("MSA") is a disease that involves progressive degeneration of multiple portions of the central nervous system that regulate the autonomic nervous system.

Several unconscious "vegetative" functions fail, such as digestion, urination, speech and swallowing mechanisms, and cardiovascular reflexes.

No one knows what causes MSA. There is no convincing evidence that in the United States the disease is inherited. No environmental toxin is known to cause it.

A currently prevalent but controversial view is that misfolded alpha-synuclein acts like a prion (an abbreviation for "proteinaceous infectious particle"). A prion is a misfolded protein that can cause misfolding of the same protein (templating), in a kind of chain reaction. The prion theory of MSA posits that misfolded alpha-synuclein is transmitted from cell to cell, induces misfolding of alpha-synuclein in target glial cells, and as a result of the glial cell pathophysiology produces central neurodegeneration as is found in MSA.

So far the theory has not been tested completely. In particular, there is no evidence for infectious spread of MSA from human to human.

According to another view, MSA reflects a form of autoimmune process where the patient's immune system attacks and destroys particular brain cells. These concepts are not mutually exclusive, since misfolded alpha-synuclein could arouse an autoimmune response.

Brain tissue from MSA patients shows abnormal accumulations of alpha-synuclein in glial cells (glial cytoplasmic inclusions, or GCIs), which are not neurons. Perhaps the accumulations interfere with the ability of glial cells to produce the nerve growth factor, glial cell line-derived neurotrophic factor (GDNF). Whether GCIs cause or are a result of the disease and the mechanisms by which alpha-synuclein accumulates in glial cells are unknown.

MSA has different forms that result in different symptoms and signs. In the parkinsonian form of MSA (MSA-P) the patient has symptoms and signs of Parkinson's disease (PD) such as slow initiation of movement, imbalance, muscular rigidity, and stooped posture. Unlike in PD, however, these problems usually do not respond well to treatment with levodopa-carbidopa, the most commonly used drug for PD, and there usually is no "pill roll" resting tremor.

In the cerebellar form of MSA (MSA-C) the patient has symptoms and signs of failure of the cerebellum, which is a part of the brain that plays an important role in coordinated movements, coherent speech, balance, and accurate gait. The tremor in cerebellar ataxia worsens with intentional movements. The patient has slurred speech and a wide-based, "drunken sailor" type gait.

Some MSA patients have both parkinsonism and cerebellar ataxia. This used to be referred to as a "mixed" form of MSA, but this term has been abandoned. Now some investigators diagnose MSA-P or MSA-C based on the main symptoms at the time of onset of the movement disorder. Others diagnose MSA-C only if there is cerebellar ataxia and no evidence of parkinsonism at any time in the disease course. By either approach, MSA-C is less common than is MSA-P.

Investigators used to equate MSA with the "Shy-Drager syndrome," which by definition involves orthostatic hypotension (OH). Others considered MSA to be an umbrella diagnosis that includes the Shy-Drager syndrome when OH figures prominently in the clinical presentation but also includes forms where signs of cerebellar atrophy or parkinsonism stand out. The eponymic term, Shy-Drager syndrome, is no longer used. Previously there also was an autonomic-dominant form of MSA, where the presenting problem was orthostatic intolerance due to OH. This designation is no longer used, although in some patients presenting with neurogenic OH, the condition evolves into MSA-P or MSA-C.

MSA is progressive and eventually lethal. The median survival time from the onset of the movement disorder (parkinsonism or cerebellar ataxia) is about a decade.

MSA differs from multiple sclerosis, which is characterized clinically by remissions and exacerbations and by relatively few changes in function of the autonomic nervous system.

MSA always involves one or more symptoms or signs of failure of the autonomic nervous system. Decreased parasympathetic nervous system (PNS) activity produces urinary retention and incontinence, constipation, and erectile failure in men.

Decreased sympathetic noradrenergic system (SNS) activity produces a fall in blood pressure when the patient stands up (orthostatic hypotension) or after a meal (post-prandial hypotension), resulting in symptoms such as dizziness, weakness, or faintness upon standing or after eating.

Symptoms and signs of brainstem neurodegeneration in MSA include particular abnormalities in eye movements (as in progressive supranuclear palsy), slurred speech, poorly coordinated swallowing, abnormal breathing (e.g., stridor), and repeated aspiration, where swallowed food goes "down the wrong pipe." These problems occasionally occur in patients with MSA who do not have orthostatic hypotension or other evidence of SNS failure.

Loss of neurons in parts of the central autonomic network probably underlie the autonomic failure in MSA. These areas include the C1 area of EPI-producing neurons in the rostral ventrolateral medulla (RVLM), which project to the sympathetic pre-ganglionic neurons in the intermediolateral columns of the spinal cord; and the A1 area of noradrenergic neurons in the caudal ventrolateral medulla (CVLM), which are part of the baroreflex arc and project to the nuclei of the hypothalamus that regulate vasopressin (AVP) release.

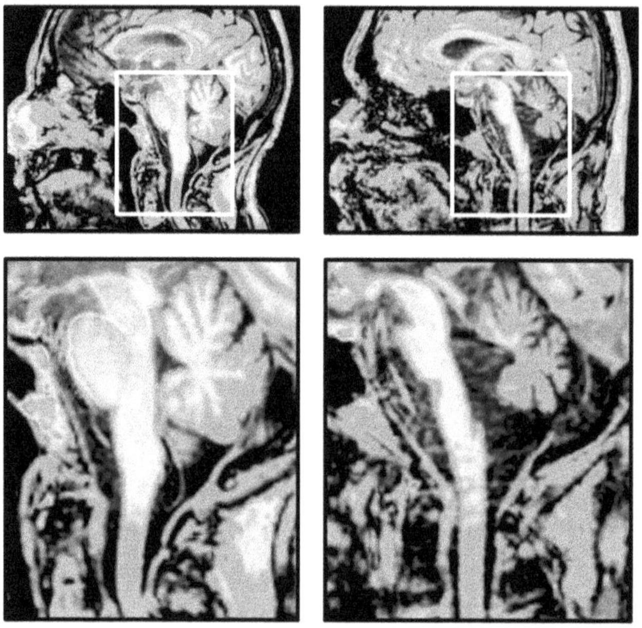

Sagittal magnetic resonance images of a healthy control (left) and a patient with multiple system atrophy (MSA). There is shrinkage of the brainstem and cerebellum in the MSA patient.

Involvement of the micturition center in the pons and Onuf's nucleus in the sacral spinal cord can account for urinary retention; and loss of neurons in the medullary pre-Bötzinger complex and raphe nuclei might play a role in sleep-related respiratory abnormalities.

Distinguishing the parkinsonian form of MSA (MSA-P) from Parkinson's disease with orthostatic hypotension (PD+OH) can be a difficult clinical diagnostic challenge. In MSA it is thought that the autonomic failure reflects loss of the ability to regulate sympathetic and parasympathetic nerve traffic appropriately, but the post-ganglionic nerves themselves are intact. This appears to be a major difference between MSA and PD+OH, in which OH is associated with a loss of sympathetic noradrenergic nerves, at least in the heart.

Because of the presence of intact sympathetic noradrenergic nerves, patients with MSA have large increases in blood pressure when they receive drugs that release norepinephrine (NE) from sympathetic nerves or inhibit the neuronal reuptake of NE. MSA patients also have large decreases in blood pressure when they receive drugs that reduce NE release from sympathetic nerves. The finding that ganglion blockade substantially decreases blood pressure in patients with MSA indicates that in MSA the problem is not so much decreased autonomic nerve traffic as failure of the brain to regulate that traffic appropriately.

During supine rest MSA patients have normal plasma levels NE and other catechols. Typically there is a failure to increase plasma NE levels normally when the patient stands up from lying down, due to baroreflex-sympathoneural failure.

In the evaluation of a patient with possible MSA the finding of urinary retention is important. Urinary retention is much more common in MSA than in Parkinson's disease with orthostatic hypotension. One reason is degeneration in a region called Onuf's nucleus, which is in the anterior horn of the sacral spinal cord. Onuf's nucleus receives descending input from the "continence center" or "micturition center" in the pons of the brainstem, and it projects to the urethral sphincter by way of the pudendal nerve. Stretch receptors in the bladder wall send afferent information to the spinal cord, and the signal is transmitted both to the brainstem and to Onuf's nucleus, completing long-distance and local negative feedback loops. It seems likely that abnormalities in both the long-distance and local loops result in the urinary retention found in MSA.

Dementia with Lewy bodies

Dementia with Lewy bodies (DLB), or Lewy body dementia (LBD), is a form of alpha-s ynucleinopathy in which cognitive dysfunction is a key part of the clinical picture. DLB is the second most common form of dementia (the first being Alzheimer's disease).

There are three core features for diagnosing DLB: (1) fluctuating cognition, attention, and alertness; (2) visual hallucinations; and (3) parkinsonism. Two of these core features should be present for a diagnosis of probable DLB, and one core feature should be present for a diagnosis of possible DLB.

There are also three suggestive features, and if there is one core feature in addition a suggestive feature, this switches the diagnosis from possible to probable DLB. The three suggestive features are: (1) dream enactment behavior, as in REM behavior disorder; (2) severe sensitivity to neuroleptic drugs (drugs used for psychoses such as schizophrenia); and (3) deficient dopamine transporter function in the basal ganglia as demonstrated by SPECT or PET imaging.

Parkinson's disease with dementia (PD+D) and Alzheimer's disease are both difficult to separate from DLB. By consensus, in PD+D, the dementia develops in the setting of already existing PD.

Two clinical characteristics may help separate DLB from Alzheimer's disease. The first is visual hallucinations, which occur commonly in DLB. The second is the clinical course. Alzheimer's disease involves a steady, progressive decline, while DLB patients have fluctuating mental status.

Clinical laboratory test that can help distinguish DLB from Alzheimer's disease include neuroimaging tests of catecholamine systems. The finding of decreased putamen 18F- DOPA-derived radioactivity would fit better with DLB than with Alzheimer's disease. DLB, as all forms of Lewy body disease, involves cardiac noradrenergic deficiency. Cardiac sympathetic neuroimaging is usually abnormal in DLB, whereas it is usually normal in Alzheimer's disease.

Seeing things? Who, me?

I once had a patient who was a retired Professor of physics at a local university. This highly intelligent and educated individual had parkinsonism, orthostatic hypotension, and cognitive impairment. How do you ask such a person if he has visual hallucinations? I put it this way: "Have you had an experience where you thought were seeing something that really wasn't there or thought you were hearing something that really wasn't there?" Here is how he answered:

> I haven't had any hallucinations—I wouldn't admit to that anyway. I do find my brain to be more creative than it used to be, in filling in the blanks, so to speak. Sometimes you'll see an image, particularly in the distance, not terribly clear, and you think it's one thing, it turns out to be another, but while you're thinking it's one thing your brain is making it look like that one thing. That phenomenon seems more pronounced to me. I've noticed my peripheral vision sometimes creates illusions, like when I'm driving it seems there's something or someone peripherally when there isn't...but no hallucinations.

Pathologically, DLB is characterized by Lewy bodies distributed widely in the brain. "Diffuse Lewy body disease" is a pathologic diagnosis, whereas DLB is a clinical diagnosis.

Stress cardiopathy

All emotions entail changes in heart functions. This fact was recognized by one of the giants in the history of medicine and physiology, William Harvey, in the 1600s.

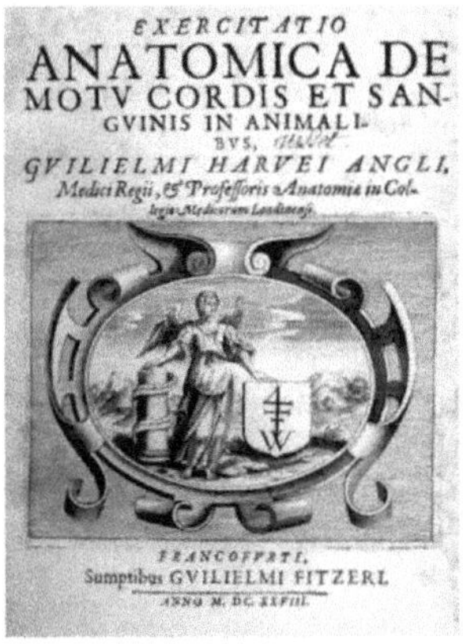
EXERCITATIO
ANATOMICA DE
MOTV CORDIS ET SAN-
GVINIS IN ANIMALI-
BVS,
GVILIELMI HARVEI ANGLI,
Medici Regii, & Professoris Anatomiæ in Col-
legio Medicorum Londinensi.

FRANCOFVRTI,
Sumptibus GVILIELMI FITZERI.
ANNO M. DC. XXVIII.

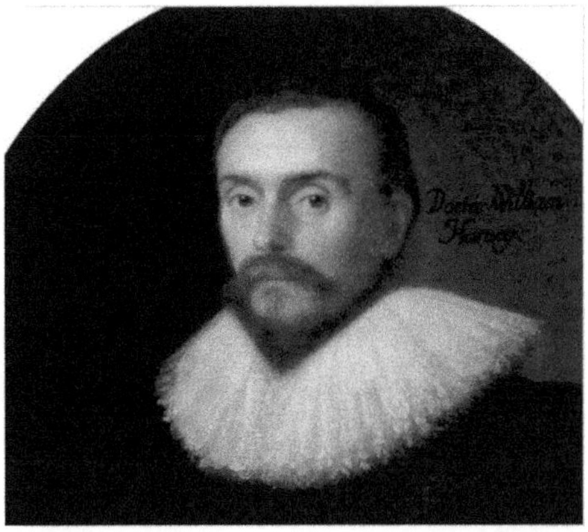

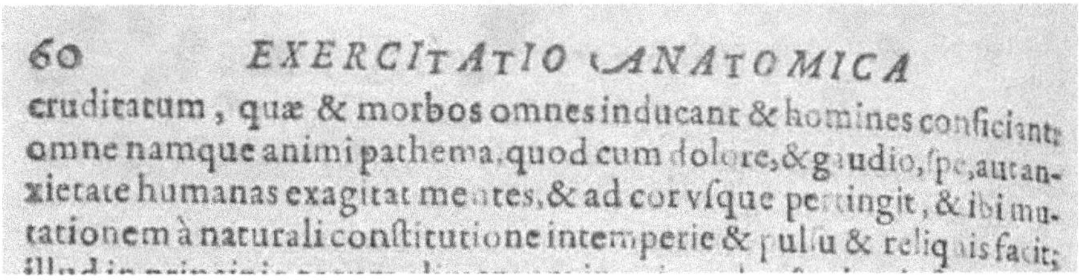
60 EXERCITATIO ANATOMICA
cruditatum, quæ & morbos omnes inducant & homines conficiant: omne namque animi pathema, quod cum dolore, & gaudio, ſpe, aut anxietate humanas exagitat mentes, & ad cor vſque pertingit, & ibi mutationem à naturali conſtitutione intemperie & pulſu & reliquis facit;

William Harvey (1578-1657) can be considered to be a founder of the fields of psychosomatic medicine and neurocardiology.

In the same book in which he described the circulation of the blood, Harvey wrote: "… for every affection of the mind that is attended with either pain or pleasure, hope or fear, is the cause of an agitation whose influence extends to the heart, and there induces change from the natural constitution, in the temperature, the pulse and the rest…"

Pathological studies about how distress can produce sudden death were not done until the past century. In 1907, about a dozen years after the discovery of the cardiovascular stimulatory effects of adrenaline, it was demonstrated that infusion of adrenaline can lead to the death of heart muscle. The heart muscle cells rupture and die of overstraining. A particular microscopic change called "contraction band necrosis" develops.

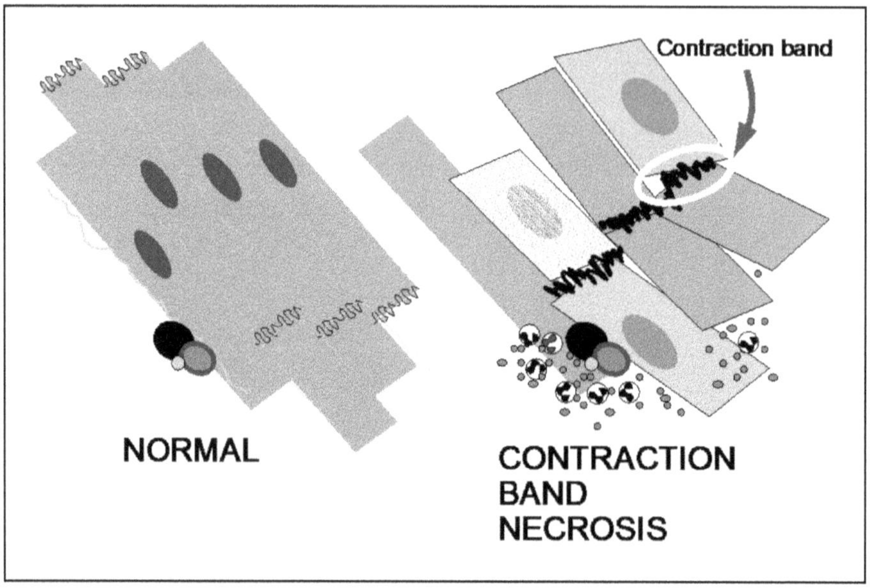

Myocardial contraction band necrosis in a histopathological finding in sudden death in the setting of severe distress.

In victims of assault who die without sufficient evidence of internal or external injury to explain the death, most have contraction band necrosis as part of the post-mortem findings. Similarly, patients who die from a stroke due to bleeding inside the brain often have contraction band necrosis (also called myocytolysis) of heart muscle cells. The extent of loss of heart muscle cells in this setting is related to the extent of increase in plasma levels of catecholamines.

Takotusubo cardiopathy

A relatively recently described form of distress-induced acute heart failure is takotsubo cardiopathy, so named because of a peculiar abnormal shape of the heart in most patients with this condition. *Takotsubo* cardiopathy has been reported to occur mainly in post-menopausal women, for reasons that are not yet completely understood. Remarkably, if the patient survives, heart muscle function can recover over a couple of weeks.

A *takotsubo* is a Japanese pottery urn used to catch octopuses. The octopus's head gets stuck in the jar (I guess, at least in this respect, octopuses are not that smart.) In *takotsubo* cardiopathy, during systole when the heart is ejecting blood, the apex of the heart balloons out while the base of the heart contracts normally. On a ventriculogram the combination of apical ballooning and basal contraction gives the appearance of a *takotsubo*. Some patients can have acute catecholamine-induced heart failure without the *takotsubo* heart shape.

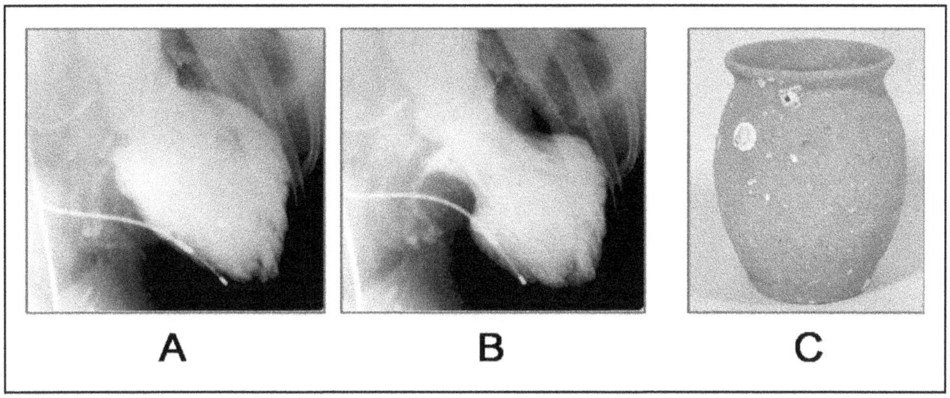

Left ventriculogram in a patient with takotsubo *cardiopathy during (A) diastole and (B) systole. There is contraction of the base of the heart but not the apex, giving the appearance of a (C)* takotsubo.

Patients with this form of stress cardiopathy have extremely high plasma EPI levels—more than 30 times normal. It seems likely that EPI levels this high are directly toxic to the heart.

The mechanisms of EPI cardiotoxicity are poorly understood. There are a few possibilities. First, at high concentrations EPI may inhibit rather than stimulate production of the second messenger adenyl cyclase, by a switch from a stimulatory to an inhibitory G-protein. Second, EPI taken up into the heart muscle cells could undergo spontaneous or enzyme-catalyzed oxidation, resulting in formation of toxic metabolites that interfere with the functions of numerous proteins required for cellular integrity. Third, EPI-mediated increased entry of ionized calcium into the cytoplasm could so contract the cells that they rupture—hence the term, "contraction band necrosis."

MANAGING DYSAUTONOMIAS

Expecting cures for dysautonomias is unrealistic in the vast majority of cases. On the other hand, there are many treatments for dysautonomias. Because there is a "universe" of dysautonomias, there is no "one size fits all" approach to management. This section emphasizes the treatments for managing dysautonomias in neurogenic orthostatic hypotension (nOH) and chronic orthostatic intolerance (COI)/POTS, because nOH is common in the geriatric age group, and COI/POTS is common in adolescents/young adults.

The key principle of management is: education first, non-drug treatments second and drug treatments third. The following text is arranged in this order.

Neurogenic Orthostatic Hypotension (nOH)

nOH can be asymptomatic.

Patients with nOH often have no symptoms when their blood pressure is low. This means it is important to have available and use a blood pressure cuff. The key measurement is the systolic blood pressure while standing.

When they do occur, symptoms of nOH can differ markedly across patients. Low blood pressure can manifest as lightheadedness or faintness but also as "coat hanger" pain, visual changes, muscle weakness, or "brain fog." Overt loss of consciousness may not happen because of the warning symptoms.

All patients with nOH should be properly educated about the basics of nOH.

Dysautonomias involving nOH include: pure autonomic failure (PAF), multiple system atrophy (MSA), and Parkinson's disease with orthostatic hypotension (PD+OH) among others.

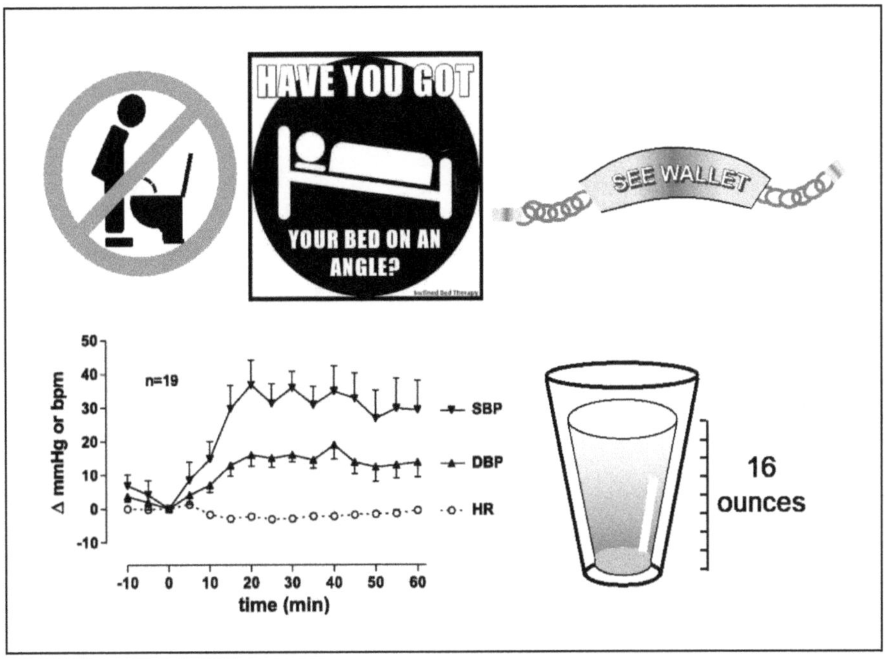

Some non-drug aspects of management of nOH. Men should urinate sitting down. The head of the bed should be elevated on blocks. Patients should wear a Medic-Alert bracelet. Drinking 16 ounces of water can raise the blood pressure.

Chronic Orthostatic Intolerance and/or Postural Tachycardia Syndrome (COI/POTS)

COI and POTS are syndromes.

Many manifestations of COI have little to do with orthostatic intolerance or excessive orthostatic tachycardia. Some of these are fatigue, "brain fog," pain (headache, temporomandibular joint syndrome, complex regional pain syndrome, abdominal pain, fibromyalgia), slow gastrointestinal transit, heat or exercise intolerance, and coat hanger phenomenon. The patient should pay attention to which of these manifestations apply, under what circumstances, and what makes things better or worse.

A substantial proportion of patients with COI/POTS have gastrointestinal symptoms and signs leading to a diagnosis of gastroesophageal reflux, slowed gastric emptying, or irritable bowel syndrome. Patients should be aware that taking a high fiber diet might worsen orthostatic intolerance by augmenting shunting of blood to the gut.

Time is a great healer. COI that comes on soon after a viral infection in an otherwise healthy person may "melt away" over many months or years. There is no convincing evidence that COI or POTS progresses to a neurodegenerative disease.

An early step in management of COI/POTS is to search carefully for common, reversible causes, such as diabetes, weight loss, prolonged bed rest, debilitating diseases, and, most importantly, medications.

In devising an individual treatment plan, it may be worthwhile to think about potential pathophysiologic mechanisms, such as low blood volume, increased splanchnic venous compliance, inefficient renal handling of salt and water, a collagen vascular disease (e.g., Ehlers-Danlos syndrome), autoimmunity, physical de-conditioning, or a primary form of hyperactivity of the sympathetic noradrenergic system. In most cases, however, pathophysiologic mechanisms remain unknown, and treatment is largely by trial and error.

Because of the debility caused by POTS, patients can get into a vicious cycle of bed rest, decreased cardiovascular and skeletal muscle tone, worsened exercise intolerance and fatigue, and more bed rest. Enrolling in an individualized exercise conditioning program can be very beneficial.

Patients with COI/POTS can feel differently from day to day without any clear reason why. This means that if a treatment is tried it may take a period of time to decide whether the treatment has helped or not.

Because of the syndromic nature of COI/POTS it may be worthwhile for the patient and clinician to target for treatment the single most troubling symptom or involved organ system.

Dysautonomias involving chronic orthostatic intolerance (COI) include autonomically mediated syncope (AMS) also known as Vasovagal Syncope (VVS), Neurocardiogenic Syncope (NCS) and postural tachycardia syndrome (POTS) among others.

Education

Morning hypotension

nOH	COI/POTS
X	

In patients with nOH the blood pressure typically is lowest in the morning, upon arising from bed. This may reflect a fall in blood volume overnight as a result of pressure natriuresis. As the day goes on, the blood pressure tends to increase. This means it would be safer for a patient with nOH to take a hot shower in the evening than morning.

The timing of taking pressor medications such as midodrine should also take this phenomenon into account. I usually have patients take 2/3 of the daily dose about an hour before trying to get out of bed in the morning and the remaining 1/3 at lunchtime (to avoid post-prandial hypotension).

In patients with COI/POTS while there may not be morning hypotension patients may struggle with fatigue and have greater difficulty with upright posture as a function of the time of day.

Risk of falls

nOH	COI/POTS
X	X

Orthostatic hypotension increases the risk of falls. That risk is magnified in patients with central neurodegeneration that manifests with a movement disorder or cognitive dysfunction. Effective management includes reviewing the housing arrangement with respect to climbing stairs. Falls are more dangerous in patients on an anti-coagulant, such as is used to prevent embolic stroke in atrial fibrillation.

Some but not all patients with COI/POTS have a history of syncope. In those patients it is helpful to determine if they experience prodromal symptoms/presyncope. If so, education about paying attention to those symptoms and preventing the fall may be helpful.

Bathrooms are dangerous

nOH	COI/POTS
X	X

Performance of the Valsalva maneuver straining at stool decreases blood pressure. It is best to avoid constipation by an appropriate bowel regimen. Constipation is treated non-specifically, with stool softeners, bulk laxatives, milk of magnesia, magnesium citrate, senna, or cascara.

Standing still while urinating can cause blood to pool in the pelvis or abdomen, and in a patient with baroreflex- sympathoneural failure whatever happens to the venous return to the heart is what happens to the blood pressure. Men with nOH should urinate while sitting on the toilet.

Patients with COI/POTS who have a history of syncope should use caution when taking a hot shower, as the heat relaxes blood vessels and may worsen orthostatic intolerance.

Heat intolerance

nOH	COI/POTS
X	X

Heat exposure relaxes blood vessels, and because of baroreflex-sympathoneural failure patients with nOH have a decreased ability to counter heat-induced decreases in blood pressure.

As mentioned previously, the combination of orthostatic, post-prandial, and heat-related hypotension is the dangerous triad I call "Florida Chinese Restaurant Syndrome."

Patients with COI/POTS often have an inability to tolerate extremes of environmental temperature. When exposed to the heat, patients with failure of the sympathetic cholinergic system may not sweat adequately to maintain the core temperature by evaporation of the sweat.

Exercise intolerance

nOH	COI/POTS
X	X

During exercise, muscle pumping can maintain the blood pressure, even as vasodilator metabolites accumulate. After exercise the blood pressure may fall. Patients with nOH should have this in mind and be ready to lie down quickly after exercising. Rather than abruptly stopping exercise it may help to gradually slow down to prevent a fall.

In patients with COI/POTS, when muscle pumping ceases after exercise the blood may pool rapidly in the legs or abdomen/pelvis as the rate of sympathetic noradrenergic nerve traffic falls to the resting rate. If the decline in nerve traffic did not balance the decline in production of byproducts of metabolism, then the blood pressure would fall after exercise. At the same time, loss of body fluid via evaporative sweating during exercise tends to decrease the blood volume. Patients therefore can feel especially unwell after exercise. It is important to stay hydrated and to avoid activities like eating a large meal immediately after exercise.

Precautions for large meals

nOH	COI/POTS
X	X

Eating a large meal shunts blood toward the gut as part of the digestive process. In a patient with nOH this shunting could come at the expense of low pressure and decreased delivery of blood to the brain. To minimize post-prandial hypotension it is advisable to take frequent, small, snack- like meals. Reducing the amounts of sugars or other carbohydrates in meals might help manage symptoms.

In people with COI/POTS who experience dizziness or lightheadedness when they stand up (orthostatic intolerance), it is usually advisable to take frequent small meals. Reducing the amounts of sugars or other carbohydrates in meals might help manage symptoms.

Precautions for supplements or OTCs

nOH	COI/POTS
X	X

Dietary supplements and over-the-counter (OTC) remedies should be reviewed carefully, because they can complicate management of nOH or increase risk. You may recall the anecdote about the MSA patient who had paroxysmal hypertension after drinking ma huang tea. Yohimbe bark contains a chemical that inhibits alpha-2 adrenoceptors and could also increase blood pressure in the setting of MSA. OTC decongestants or vasoconstrictor eyedrops might increase blood pressure in a patient with baroreflex-sympathoneural failure.

Precautions for air travel

nOH	COI/POTS
X	X

Air travel poses several risks in nOH patients. These include standing relatively motionless on line for TSA security checks. Depending on the severity of nOH, a medical escort may be needed. As noted previously, the bathroom in a jet is an especially dangerous place. I don't know if low cabin pressure (which decreases the amount of oxygen in the air) poses a threat.

In patients with COI/POTS sitting motionless for long periods in a jet may worsen symptoms. During the flight it may be helpful to get up out of the seat periodically to walk as muscle pumping helps to maintain venous return during orthostasis. Patients may find it helpful to load with salt and fluids prior to the flight.

Precautions for surgery/anesthesia

nOH	COI/POTS
X	X

During surgery under general anesthesia there can be large swings in blood pressure because of baroreflex-sympathoneural failure in patients with nOH. Patients with COI/POTS may experience exaggerated hemodynamic variation while under general anesthesia. In patients who require prolonged hospitalization following surgery early mobilization is helpful to prevent deconditioning.

Cardiac ectopy

nOH	COI/POTS
X	

There is an increased likelihood of cardiac ectopy in nOH. Blood pressure may fall excessively when there is a change in heart rhythm, manifesting with palpitations.

Non-Drug Treatments

Exercise and rehabilitation medicine

nOH	COI/POTS
X	X

Patients with nOH in the setting of progressive central neurodegeneration should stay as active physically as possible and have a home exercise program. Physical medicine and rehabilitation efforts have the goal of maximizing mobility and minimizing the risk of aspiration.

In patients with COI/POTS, maintaining good muscle tone in the anti-gravity muscles of the buttocks, thighs, and calves maximizes the efficiency of muscle pumping to maintain venous return to the heart during orthostasis. Exercise improves the ability to increase cardiac output. Moreover, in chronic, debilitating disorders it is important for the patient to regain a sense of at least some control over the situation.

Patients with COI sometimes benefit markedly from an individualized exercise training program. Some reasonable exercises in patients with COI/POTS include anti-gravity muscle resistance training, swimming, or graded exercise training. Often, however, the training does not eliminate the sense of fatigue. It might help to have small amounts of exercise daily, even for only 5-10 minutes. Preventing deconditioning is an important aim for COI/POTS patients.

Compression garments

nOH	COI/POTS
X	X

Because of the baroreflex failure attending OH from chronic autonomic failure, decreases in venous return to the heart are translated into decreased blood pressure. When a person stands up, blood tends to pool in the abdomen, pelvis, and legs.

In nOH the problem is less with the veins than with the arteries and arterioles, the blood vessels that carry oxygen-rich blood under high pressure to the organs and limbs. Wearing thigh-high compression stockings is inconvenient and may not be particularly beneficial in the management of nOH.

Inflation of an abdominal binder (which resembles a huge blood pressure cuff) squeezes blood out of the abdomen towards the chest and increases venous return to the heart. In a patient with baroreflex-sympathoneural failure this should raise the blood pressure. An automated abdominal binder has been under development for several to mitigate OH but is not yet commercially available.

Compression hose or other compression garments tend to decrease the amount of pooling of blood in abdominal and pelvic veins when a person stands. This can decrease leakage of fluid from the veins into the tissues and decrease leg swelling. In patients with veins that fill up or leak excessively during standing, compression garments can improve toleration of prolonged standing. In COI patients a "step-in" abdominal binder (e.g., a doubled bicycle leotard or Spanx™) may be more efficient than compression stockings, by limiting orthostatic blood pooling in the abdomen and pelvis.

Counter-maneuvers

nOH	COI/POTS
X	X

Counter-maneuvers can temporarily maintain blood pressure during upright posture. These include tightening the buttocks, thighs, and calves (recall the "pretzel legs" sign). In an exercise training program, it may be valuable to focus on maximizing the tone of anti-gravity muscles (e.g., rowing machine, swimming).

At the time of an acute episode, isometric counter-maneuvers such as leg crossing and tightening the buttocks can temporarily maintain consciousness in patients with nOH or COI/POTS.

High salt intake

nOH	COI/POTS
X	X

Normally when a person takes in a high salt diet the kidneys increase the amount of salt in the urine, and this limits the increase in blood volume. After a few days of the same salt intake, the rate of sodium excretion equals the rate of intake. For a high salt diet to increase body fluid volume effectively, drugs that promote retention of sodium by the kidneys, such as fludrocortisone, are usually required.

In patients with COI/POTS doctors usually recommend a high salt diet with electrolyte drinks.

Elevation of the head of the bed

nOH	COI/POTS
X	

In patients with nOH, elevation of the head of the bed on blocks at night decreases the severity of supine hypertension and improves the ability to tolerate standing up in the morning.

Water drinking

nOH	COI/POTS
X	X

A sometimes very effective tactic to increase blood pressure in patients with nOH is to drink 16 ounces of water. There is an "osmopressor response," in which ingested water without solute acts in the gut or liver to increase sympathetic noradrenergic system outflow. The sensors evoking the response are still unknown.

Water bolus drinking also helps prevent syncope and improve orthostatic intolerance in patients with COI/POTS.

CPAP + heat

nOH	COI/POTS
X	

A substantial proportion of patients with nOH have obstructive sleep apnea and are treated with continuous positive airway pressure (CPAP). By increasing intrathoracic pressure, CPAP may tend to decrease venous return to the heart and therefore decrease blood pressure. CPAP combined with a warming blanket to relax blood vessels might ameliorate nocturnal supine hypertension.

Drug Treatments

Fludrocortisone

nOH	COI/POTS
X	X

Fludrocortisone (Florinef™) is a man-made type of drug called a salt-retaining steroid, or mineralocorticoid. The drug closely resembles the body's main salt-retaining steroid, aldosterone.

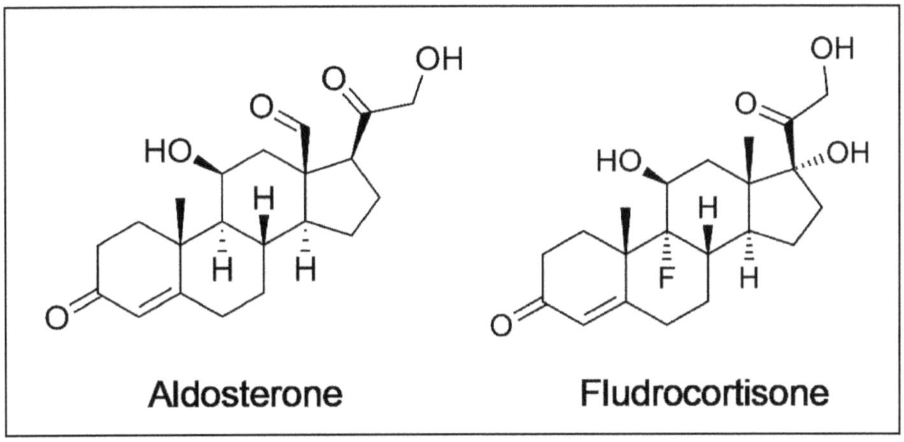

The chemical structure of fludrocortisone closely resembles that of aldosterone, the body's main salt-retaining steroid.

In order for fludrocortisone to work the drug must be taken with a high-salt diet. A target urinary sodium excretion rate is 200 mEq per day.

Fludrocortisone forces the kidneys to retain sodium in exchange for potassium. Water follows the sodium, and so fludrocortisone is thought to increase the blood volume. The patient gains "fluid weight," and blood pressure increases. Because of the tendency of fludrocortisone to waste potassium, fludrocortisone can cause a fall in the serum potassium level. Patients taking fludrocortisone should have periodic checks of their serum potassium level, and if it is low they should take a potassium supplement.

Fludrocortisone treatment increases the blood pressure regardless of the patient's posture. The increased blood pressure when the patient is standing may come at the cost of supine hypertension.

In some patients with COI/POTS, treatment with fludrocortisone coupled with a high salt diet can produce improvement; however, in other patients there is no improvement. Perhaps this treatment is effective only in patients who have low blood volume or decreased ability of the kidneys to reabsorb filtered sodium, but there is little relevant research literature. For fludrocortisone to work, the drug should be taken with a high salt diet. A simple sign of drug effect is that the patient gains "fluid weight."

In patients with COI/POTS fludrocortisone helps to increase blood volume, increase blood pressure, and alleviate salt wasting.

Midodrine

nOH	COI/POTS
X	X

When a person stands up, the sympathetic noradrenergic system is activated reflexively, the chemical messenger norepinephrine (NE) is released from the sympathetic nerves in blood vessel walls, the NE binds to alpha-adrenoceptors in the blood vessel walls, and the stimulation of the alpha-adrenoceptors causes the blood vessels to constrict (vasoconstriction), increasing the blood pressure. Midodrine is a vasoconstrictor that works by stimulating alpha-adrenoceptors in blood vessel walls.

In patients with orthostatic hypotension related to a loss of sympathetic noradrenergic nerves, there is little NE to release. In this situation, the blood vessels become supersensitive ("denervation supersensitivity"), perhaps by the alpha-adrenoceptors accumulating on the surface of the cells in blood vessel walls. In patients with denervation supersensitivity midodrine can be especially effective in raising the blood pressure.

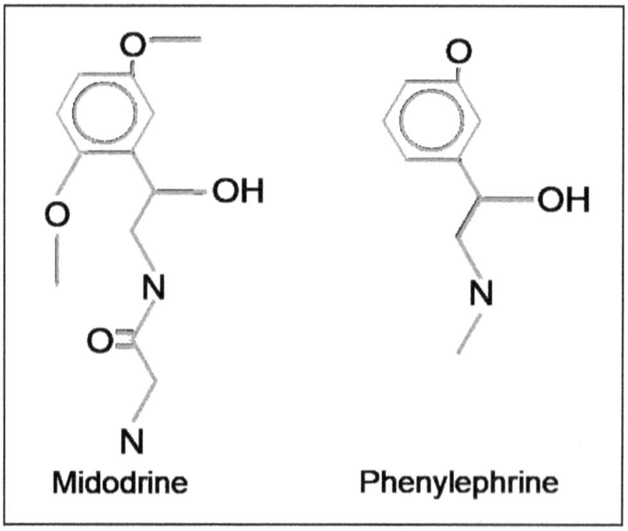

The orally active alpha-adrenoceptor agonist midodrine is closely related structurally to the classic alpha-1 adrenoceptor agonist phenylephrine.

In patients with sympathetic denervation taking midodrine around the clock may desensitize the alpha-adrenoceptors. It is reasonable to try taking midodrine early in the morning before getting up and then perhaps at lunchtime to avoid post-prandial hypotension but not to take it later in the day, so that by the next morning the drug has worn off and the alpha-adrenoceptors are maximally responsive.

Stimulation of alpha-adrenoceptors can worsen symptoms of prostate problems. Alpha-1 adrenoceptor blockers are effective in treating benign prostatic hypertrophy (BPH), but alpha-1 adrenoceptors blockers interfere with midodrine's effects.

In patients with COI/POTS midodrine helps to tighten blood vessels, increase blood pressure and prevent fainting.

Droxidopa (L-DOPS)

nOH	COI/POTS
X	X

L-Dihydroxyphenylserine (L-DOPS, droxidopa, Northera™) is an amino acid. It is very closely related chemically to L-dihydroxyphenylalanine (Levodopa, L- DOPA), which is an effective drug to treat Parkinson's disease. L-DOPA works by being converted in the brain to the catecholamine dopamine. L-DOPS works by being converted to the closely related catecholamine norepinephrine (NE).

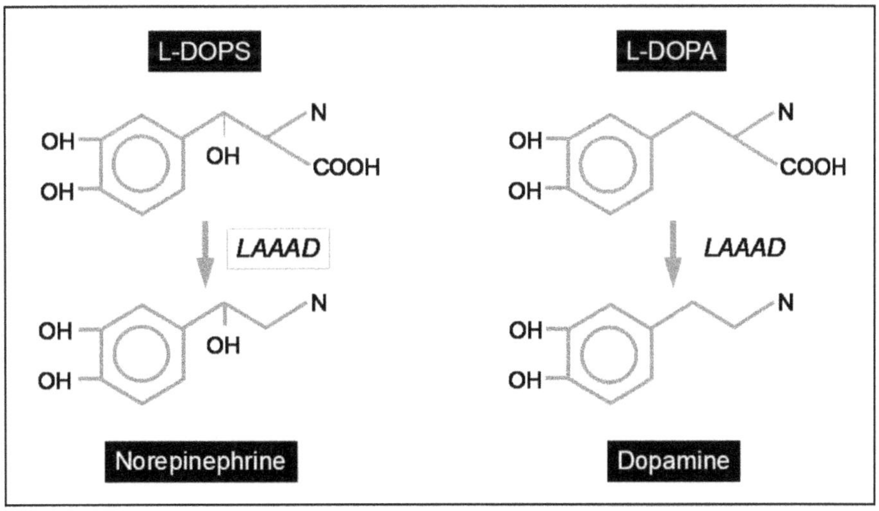

L-DOPS is converted to norepinephrine like L-DOPA is converted to dopamine.

L-DOPS is a neutral amino acid and as such is taken up into all cells via the neutral amino acid transporter. In cells of the gut, liver, kidneys, and other organs that contain abundant L- aromatic-amino-acid decarboxylase (LAAAD), L-DOPS is converted efficiently to NE. This means that L-DOPS can provide NE even in the absence of sympathetic nerves.

Because L-DOPS is a NE pro-drug, L-DOPS administration leads indirectly to stimulation of alpha- adrenoceptors in blood vessel walls, causing the vessels to constrict and increasing the blood pressure.

A potential problem with using L-DOPS to treat orthostatic hypotension in patients with Parkinson's disease is that the patients usually are being treated at the same time with a combination of L-DOPA and carbidopa. The carbidopa interferes with the conversion of L-DOPA to dopamine. Since carbidopa does not enter the brain, the combination results in increased delivery of DOPA to the brain and increased production of dopamine. Carbidopa also interferes with the conversion of L-DOPS to NE. This might blunt the hoped-for increase in blood pressure by L-DOPS treatment; however, it appears that doses of levodopa/carbidopa used clinically the amount of LAAAD inhibition is too small to prevent the L-DOPS-induced increase in blood pressure.

In patients with COI/POTS droxidopa helps to tighten blood vessels, increase blood pressure, and produce vasoconstriction.

Pyridostigmine

nOH	COI/POTS
X	X

Pyridostigmine (Mestinon™) works by inhibiting acetylcholinesterase, the enzyme that breaks down acetylcholine (ACh). ACh is the chemical messenger that is responsible for transmission of autonomic nerve impulses in ganglia. By attenuating the breakdown of ACh, pyridostigmine is thought to increase activity of the sympathetic nervous system and improve orthostatic hypotension.

Because pyridostigmine also increases activity of the parasympathetic nervous system, the drug can increase salivation and stimulate gastrointestinal or urinary bladder contractions. There may be psychological changes because of actions of the drug in the brain. By increasing activity of the sympathetic cholinergic system pyridostigmine can increase sweat production.

In patient with COI/POTS pyridostigmine helps to increase blood pressure.

Beta-adrenoceptor blockade

nOH	COI/POTS
	X

Norepinephrine and epinephrine produce their effects by binding to specific receptors, adrenoceptors, on target cells such as heart muscle cells.

Beta-blockers interfere with this binding. Drugs that act at beta-adrenoceptors are often grouped in terms of whether they are "selective" for beta-1 adrenoceptors or are "non-selective," meaning they block the other types of beta- adrenoceptors as well. In patients with COI/POTS beta-blockers help decrease heart rate, decrease blood pressure, decrease epinephrine effects and prevent fainting.

In patients with autonomically mediated syncope and high levels of epinephrine in the bloodstream, the epinephrine stimulates beta-2 adrenoceptors on blood vessels in skeletal muscle. This relaxes the blood vessels and decreases the resistance to blood flow. Blood may then be shunted away from the brain and towards the skeletal muscle, contributing to lightheadedness or loss of consciousness. In such patients, non-selective beta-adrenoceptor blockers might be preferable to selective blockers. There are no approved drugs that block beta-2 adrenoceptors selectively.

In patients with COI/POTS the value of treatment with beta-adrenoceptor blockers will depend on whether the rapid pulse rate when the patient stands up reflects a primary or compensatory response. If the rapid pulse rate were a compensation for another problem, such as low blood volume, then blocking that compensation would not help. If the rapid pulse rate were the result of an excessive rate of sympathetic nerve traffic to the heart, or there were a high intrinsic heart rate, then a beta-adrenoceptor blocker might help.

Beta-blockers should be used with caution in COI/POTS patients with mast cell activation disorder, as these drugs can elicit mast cell degranulation.

Benzodiazepines

nOH	COI/POTS
	X

In patients with COI/POTS benzodiazepines such as alprazolam (=Xanax™) or clonazepam (=Klonopin™) help increase a sense of calmness, improve sleep, and attenuate epinephrine release. Benzodiazepines may be helpful in patients with mast cell activation disorders as they have mast cell stabilizing effects.

Clonidine

nOH	COI/POTS
	X

In patients with COI/POTS clonidine (=Catapres™) helps to decrease blood pressure and improve sleep. Clonidine stimulates alpha-2 adrenoceptors. Stimulation of alpha-2 adrenoceptors in the brain decreases the rate of sympathetic nerve traffic, and stimulation of alpha-2 adrenoceptors on sympathetic nerves decreases the amount of release of the chemical messenger norepinephrine from the nerves. Even though clonidine stimulates a type of alpha- adrenoceptor, the drug normally decreases the blood pressure.

There are several uses of clonidine in the diagnosis and treatment of dysautonomias. In the clonidine suppression test, clonidine is used to separate high blood pressure due to increased sympathetic nervous system activity from high blood pressure due to a tumor that produces catecholamines—pheochromocytoma.

In patients with long-term high blood pressure (hypertension) due to excessive release of norepinephrine from sympathetic nerves (hypernoradrenergic hypertension), clonidine can be very effective in lowering the blood pressure. Clonidine is also effective in treating withdrawal from some addictive drugs.

Clonidine may attenuate the large swings in blood pressure that are associated with baroreflex failure.

Clonidine often causes drowsiness and dry mouth. The side effects may limit its clinical use.

Amphetamines

nOH	COI/POTS
X	X

Amphetamines are chemicals that resemble the drug dextro-amphetamine (d-amphetamine). They share a particular chemical structure (alpha-methyl-phenylethylamine).

Amphetamines are indirectly acting sympathomimetic amines. They produce their effects at least partly by increasing delivery of norepinephrine to its receptors, both in the brain and outside the brain.

By way of effects in the brain, amphetamines increase the state of arousal and attention, prevent or reverse fatigue, decrease appetite, and at high doses increase the rate and depth of breathing. They also increase blood pressure, probably by multiple mechanisms in the brain and periphery.

Pseudoephedrine (Sudafed™) is structurally a mirror image (stereoisomer) of ephedrine. This difference changes the properties of the drug and produces much less central nervous system stimulation. By releasing norepinephrine from sympathetic nerve terminals in the mucous membranes of the nasal airways, pseudoephedrine tightens blood vessels, making them less leaky and thereby relieving nasal congestion.

In a laboratory pseudoephedrine can be converted easily to other amphetamines that are abused drugs. This is why over-the-counter sales of pseudoephedrine are now restricted. Methylphenidate (Ritalin™), another sympathomimetic amine, is used commonly to treat attention deficit-hyperactivity disorder.

In patients with COI/POTS amphetamines help to tighten blood vessels and increase alertness. Amphetamines should be used sparingly because of the potential for tolerance and dependence.

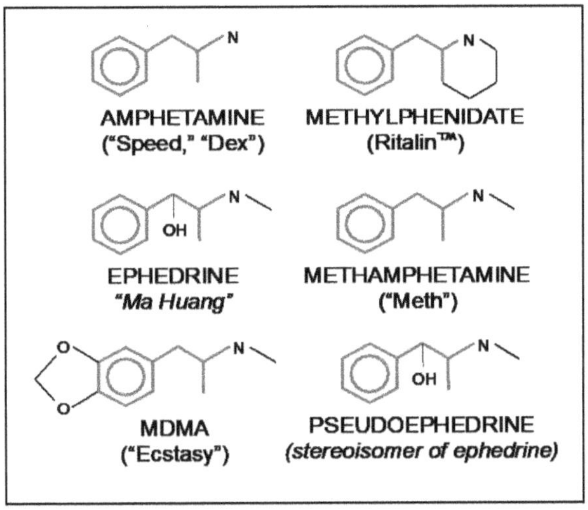

Some amphetamines. Amphetamines resemble catecholamines but have a methyl group at the alpha carbon on the hydrocarbon tail and lack adjacent hydroxyl groups on the benzene ring. Amphetamines are not catechols.

Somatostatin

nOH	COI/POTS
X	X

Somatostatin (Octreotide™) is a hormone that inhibits the release of another hormone, growth hormone, from the pituitary gland at the base of the brain. Somatostatin can tighten blood vessels, especially in the gastrointestinal tract, and raise the blood pressure of patients with orthostatic hypotension. The drug must be injected, and it is expensive.

SSRIs

nOH	COI/POTS
X	X

Selective serotonin reuptake inhibitors (SSRIs) inhibit a key process that is required for inactivating and recycling the chemical messenger serotonin. The process is reuptake of released serotonin back into the nerve terminals.

SSRIs are widely used to treat depression, anxiety, and other psychiatric or emotional problems. Patients with nOH often are treated with SSRIs. This class of drugs exerts relatively little effects on autonomic functions.

Drugs that directly or indirectly increase occupation of serotonin receptors can under some circumstances produce a syndrome of confusion, twitching, diarrhea, headache, and evidence of sympathetic activation.

In patients with COI/POTS SSRIs help to improve mood and allay anxiety.

A special word of caution is in order about the treatment of teenagers with dysautonomia who are depressed: Monoamine reuptake blockers have been statistically associated with an increased risk of suicide.

Intravenous saline

nOH	COI/POTS
	X

Inability to tolerate prolonged standing can result from low blood volume, excessive pooling of blood in the veins of the legs, pelvis, or abdomen during standing, or exit of fluid from the blood vessels into the tissues (extravasation).

In these situations, IV infusion of physiological saline solution can temporarily improve the ability to tolerate standing up. IV saline infusion can also be useful for diagnostic purposes. Some patients with COI/POTS benefit from IV saline infusion given a few times per week by way of a permanent intravenous catheter. The clinician must weigh the potential benefit against the not insubstantial risks of infection and intravascular clotting.

IDEAS FOR THE FUTURE

In the study of autonomic medicine there are many ideas which are worthy of greater investigation for the future. In the full online text several ideas are suggested. This abbreviated section highlights two of the most important ideas; The extended autonomic nervous system (EAS) and flipping the clinic.

The Extended Autonomic System (EAS)

It is time to extend the meaning of "autonomic."

Almost exactly a century ago John Newport Langley defined the autonomic nervous system (ANS) as consisting of three parts—the sympathetic nervous system, the parasympathetic nervous system (PNS), and the enteric nervous system (ENS). These purely efferent systems would transmit neuronal signals to body organs via ganglia.

Discoveries in the intervening century have rendered Langley's definition obsolete, for three reasons. First, a variety of neuroendocrine and autocrine/paracrine systems also mediate automatic, unconscious, involuntary activities in the body's "inner world." Second, components of the ANS interact complexly and dynamically with the immune and inflammatory systems—an area that seems particular relevant to post-infectious disorders of regulation after viral illnesses. Third, the ANS is regulated via anatomic and neurotransmitter centers and pathways in the brain—the central autonomic network (CAN), which not only modulates autonomic outflows but also receives and integrates afferent signals from the periphery.

After Walter B. Cannon extended on Langley's ANS to include a hormonal component, here called the sympathetic adrenergic system (SAS), many additional neuroendocrine systems have been described that figure prominently in regulation of internal variables.

Examples are the hypothalamic-pituitary-adrenocortical (HPA) system, the renin-angiotensin-aldosterone system (RAS), and the arginine vasopressin (AVP)/anti-diuretic hormone (ADH) system. There also are autocrine-paracrine systems such as the renal DOPA-dopamine system, locally released and acting nitric oxide in response to parasympathetic nervous system (PNS)-mediated acetylcholine release, endogenous opiates, co- transmitters, and a large array of cytokines.

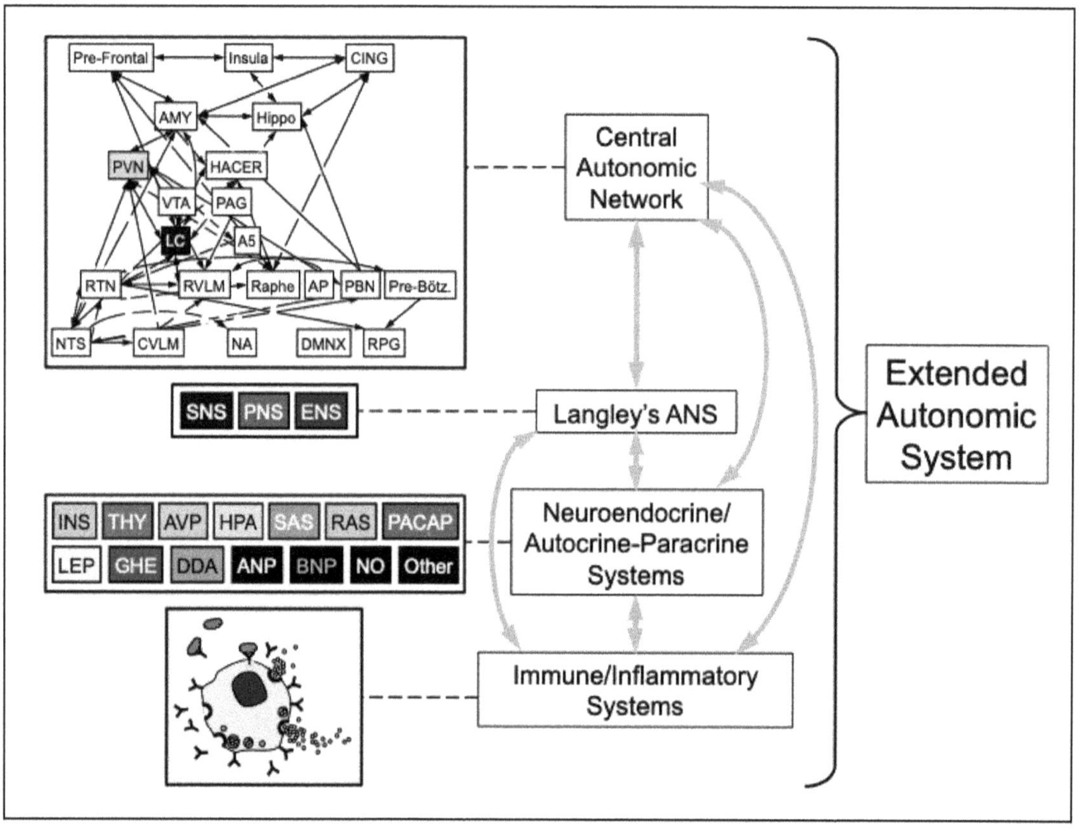

The extended autonomic system (EAS) has 4 components—Langley's ANS, neuroendocrine systems such as the sympathetic adrenergic system (SAS), immune/inflammatory systems, and the central autonomic network.

Also in the century since Langley proposed the ANS a variety of immune/inflammatory systems have been described, including the cholinergic anti-inflammatory and catecholamine-related inflammasomal systems.

Reciprocal influences among the four components of the EAS (6 combinations of interactions) set the stage for feedback loops that maintain homeostasis and for feed-forward alterations in input-output curves that underlie allostasis.

The EAS concept provides a framework for generating testable hypotheses related to the pathophysiology and pathophysiology-based treatment of a wide variety of complex, multi-system disorders of regulation.

Flipping the Clinic

The term, "flip the clinic," refers to an initiative by the Robert Wood Johnson Foundation (RWJF). RWJF considers this to be less a full-fledged program than a "conversation" in progress.

Flipping the clinic is an attempt to achieve two goals. The first goal is to enable healthcare providers to improve the ways they communicate with patients and support them better during and between office visits. The second goal is to empower patients, family, and caregivers to be more informed and engaged in their own health and health care.

The notion of flipping the clinic draws inspiration from Sal Khan, founder of Khan Academy, the well-known not-for-profit organization that aims to offer "free world-class education" online, through an extensive library of videos and lectures as well as interactive challenges and assessments. Khan Academy has sought to "flip" the classroom.

From a scientific point of view, flipping the clinic will be especially valuable for patients with multi-system disorders of regulation, such as dysautonomias. A system of education, lifestyle adjustments, support groups, and internet-based outcomes research can be compared with the standard medical practice models, in terms of both cost-efficiency and patient satisfaction.

I hope this book is a step in that direction.

www.ingramcontent.com/pod-product-compliance
Lightning Source LLC
Chambersburg PA
CBHW041748220926
51847CB00013B/138
* 9 7 8 1 9 3 8 8 4 2 6 7 2 *